Practical techniques that work at the level of the mind-
yoga, and qi gong, are growing in popularity as tools for
many people, these practices are still shrouded in a mys
which often emphasizes their peculiarities and any de
Perhaps this is most applicable to hypnosis, which has an
a strange and complicated phenomenon. In this book. Dr. Burke has delivered a simple but
thorough description of the mind-body technique of self-hypnosis, which cuts through the
stereotype associated with hypnosis and provides a clear understanding of the process and
simple instructions for practicing it. His clinical experience with self-hypnosis is evident
throughout the text and this is particularly helpful in conveying the principles and basic techniques in a very personable manner. It is a very useful handbook.

—SAT BIR S. KHASALA, Ph.D.,
Instructor in Medicine, Harvard Medical School

Self-Hypnosis presents an easily learned approach that you can use to become more focused,
creative, and effective in achieving your goals. Adam Burke, Ph.D., makes a strong case for
learning to make use of our human capability to move easily between our normal waking
state of consciousness and other states of consciousness. Burke guides you through a variety of simple, self-hypnosis exercises. He encourages you to use these exercises to serve the
values that you hold most dearly. *Self-Hypnosis* is a practical book that also inspires.

—CHERYL KOOPMAN, Ph.D.,
Associate Professor, Department of Psychiatry and Behavioral Sciences,
Stanford University

Dr. Adam Burke has written a wonderfully empowering guide to self-hypnosis. Whether
you have specific problems in which you want improvement or simply want to learn to
quiet and expand your mind, this book can help you.

—DANA ULLMAN, MPII,
author of *Homeopathy A–Z* and
Homeopathic Medicines for Children and Infants and
co-author of *Everybody's Guide to Homeopathic Medicines*

Beginning with the importance of our beliefs, Burke outlines a blueprint on which to
base a practice of self-hypnosis. In this well-organized and comprehensive practical work-
book, he provides a guided tour through the architecture of our soma and psyche, offer-
ing a new tool for self-discovery. This is an immense resource for the individual interested
in embarking on their own journey as well as for the integrative case provider to share with
appropriate patients. Self-hypnosis promises to become an increasingly important mind-
body medicine modality.

—DONALD I. ABRAMS, M.D.,
Professor of Medicine, Hematology-Oncology,
University of California, San Francisco

SELF-HYPNOSIS

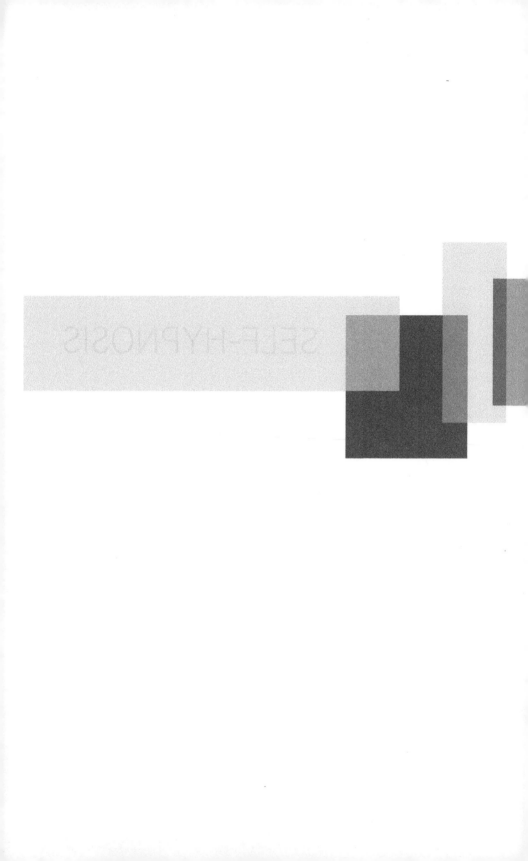

SELF-HYPNOSIS

New Tools for Deep and Lasting Transformation

Adam Burke, Ph.D., MHP, Lac

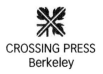

CROSSING PRESS
Berkeley

All rights reserved. Published in the United States by
Crossing Press, an imprint of the Crown Publishing Group,
a division of Random House, Inc., New York.
www.crownpublishing.com
www.tenspeed.com

Crossing Press and the Crossing Press colophon are
registered trademarks of Random House, Inc.

Library of Congress Cataloging-in-Publication Data
Burke, Adam.
Self-hypnosis: new tools for deep and lasting
transformation / Adam Burke.
        p. cm.
Includes index.
1. Autogenic training I. Title.

RC499.A8B876 2004
615.8'5122—dc22   2003067476

ISBN-13: 978-1-58091-136-8 (alk. paper)

Printed in the United States of America

Design by Catherine Jacobes Design
Cover photo by Getty Images

14 13 12 11 10 9 8 7 6

First Edition

contents

preface

Self-hypnosis is a powerful tool for promoting healing, growth, and transformation. It works by activating a creative state of mind and body where new learning can occur effectively, almost effortlessly. Once awakened this creative space can help provide you with the knowledge and energy you need to succeed in life, helping to build new beliefs and to focus action. Through regular practice, you will find a richer life unfolding naturally, with deeper friendships, faster healing, increased income, improved concentration and learning, enhanced sports performance, whatever you seek.

The process is simple, it does not take much time, and the results can be truly incredible. Basically all that you need is a goal, a few minutes to focus quietly, and a simple process for realizing success. Individuals who are ready for change will find *Self-Hypnosis* to be an essential learning resource. This book provides a palette of techniques for working with personal goals and life dreams. By following the methods provided you can quickly begin making progress on your goals and feel more in control of your life and your destiny. Working with these tools can empower anyone to move toward his or her potential more confidently and more powerfully. The only limit is the size of your dreams.

Regarding the ideas in this book, although the theories about hypnosis and how it works are diverse and not uncontroversial, I have elected to present a specific model of mind, body, and transformation that makes sense to me and produces results for my clients and students. It has evolved over the years based on my work with acupuncture as a form of energy medicine, meditation systems, and many varieties of hypnotic techniques. The result is a vision of hypnosis as a tool to modify belief, working with the subtle architecture of psyche and soma, opening us to a more aligned and potent power within. In time all ideas evolve and change. It is hoped that the ideas and tools presented here will offer food for thought and, more important, tools for lasting and gratifying change. Good luck and enjoy the journey.

self-hypnosis and TRANSFORMATION

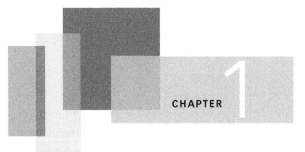

life's potential

Self-hypnosis is a simple, practical tool for transforming beliefs. Why is that important? The beliefs we hold about self, others, and the world influence every single experience we have. If we believe we are not smart enough or that we are unattractive, that the world is not safe, or that we are not loved by other people, then our life becomes very limited, very constricted. On the other hand, if we believe that we are worthy, that the world is good, and that we are loved by others, then our life expands. It is really quite simple.

Beyond Limits

Our positive beliefs inspire us. They allow us to embrace dreams, to harness healing energy, to have hope and confidence, and to take empowered action. Positive beliefs strengthen and encourage us; perhaps we can say they liberate us. Certainly both types of beliefs, positive and negative, are within us. The thing to remember is that we always have a choice about which beliefs will constitute the core of our reality. If we want to be happy, if we hope to live a powerful life, the appropriate choice becomes clear. To experience deep healing and high happiness it is imperative that we act to reduce our limiting beliefs and to replace them with powerful new positive beliefs. We all possess the potential for an incredible life journey. Such a life

1

begins and ends with empowered beliefs. If we can learn to work more intentionally with our beliefs then we will possess a key to achieving the greatest life possible.

The Healing Journey

When we heal our beliefs, those transformed beliefs can begin to heal us. The task of belief transformation, however, is not necessarily an easy one. It is challenging because of a number of internal mechanisms that are designed to protect our past beliefs and to resist the introduction of new information that might alter them. To succeed in the process of transforming and empowering new beliefs we need to strategically address those protective mechanisms.

One approach is to cultivate new beliefs through self-hypnosis. How does that work? It is a process by which we take in ideas, in the form of specifically structured visual or verbal information, and plant them at a deep level within our mind and body. When we work at this deep mind-body level we experience the information as its own reality, just as dreams are experienced as a reality. Self-hypnosis helps us to sink below the tangle of voices that say our dream is too big, that we will not succeed, that no one has ever done that before. It helps us to sink below those internal vigilance mechanisms that are designed to hold us in place by reducing receptivity to new information and new possibilities. Here we can explore new possibilities. With self-hypnosis we can enter a place of hope. The gates are open. Here our true vision can awaken, and we can wisely craft the life of our dreams.

Self-hypnosis gives us more access to life's potential. It can be used for working on relationship issues, body and health concerns, addictions, athletic performance, self-image, anxiety, public speaking, earning more money, improving one's sex life, experiencing greater courage, getting better grades, passing exams, finding a career; the list is endless. If your beliefs affect an issue, beliefs about yourself, the world, or life, then self-hypnosis can help. Self-hypnosis goes to the root level of our perceptions about life providing the requisite nourishment and vital energy necessary for deep change to occur. It is a simple tool that gives us a way to become the person we were born to be.

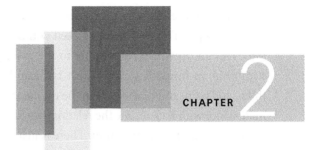

the power of belief

If we can heal our beliefs, our beliefs can heal us. Beliefs play a critical role in the successes and failures in our life. As such it is wise for us to understand the nature of our beliefs. In the simplest sense beliefs are ideas we hold about ourselves, others, and the world. These ideas are quite powerful. They help us to know who we are, what we are capable of, and what life can offer us. As such they become a foundation of our self-identity and a basis for our expectations and our dreams. We are, to a large extent, what we believe we are. The world is, to a large extent, what we believe it is.

The Nature of Self

The relationship between belief and self-identity is very important. To understand it we should begin by considering what constitutes self. Meditations on this topic are probably as old as human awareness. From the philosophies of the ancient East to the modern cognitive sciences, the phenomena of the self has often been described as consisting of two distinct expressions. One aspect is our existential self. This is the undifferentiated self, which has no labels and no inner narrative. It is just pure awareness and pure consciousness. This would be like the self of the very, very young infant. The newborn lives with us in the world of politics, social class, race, and religion, but it has little self-conscious identification with those concepts. This new being is a self without personal history or opinions. It is an organism responding to the raw signals of inner and outer stimuli in an immediate and direct fashion. It senses hunger, pleasure, thirst, and pain, and it responds in the moment. This responding is an intimate dance with nature, like the relationship of wind and wave. There is no forethought and no expectation. There is just the responding and returning. It is as Jesus said, that we must be as innocent as children to enter the kingdom of heaven. The experience of that pure self is the return to the Garden.

Such natural innocence, however, does not endure. For in addition to this existential self we also have a social self, which begins to show itself in the first few months of life. Before we are two years old, we have a basic sense of gender, right and wrong, ownership, and many other fundamental self understandings. This social self is fashioned through our interactions with others and the world. This is the self with labels and narrative and history. Our social self is a collection of beliefs about class, gender, race, aptitude, attractiveness, age, and all the rest, coming together to form a somewhat coherent body of beliefs. These beliefs are a repository of complex interrelated meanings, a mass of data we have acquired about people, places, ideas, things, processes, and events. As a personal archive our beliefs help us to determine whether the people, places, and things we experience are safe or unsafe, useful or irrelevant, desirable or undesirable, beyond our reach or a part of our destiny. They help us to know how to respond. In this way our social self, with its array of beliefs, becomes the interface between perceiving and responding, a highly personal filter in our interpreting, understanding, and decision-making processes, an ever-present mediator of the experiences of life.

The Problem with Beliefs

In essence, our beliefs provide prepackaged information. They remind us of how we feel about things and shade our sense of the way things should be. If we believe we are not good at something, we avoid doing it. If we believe people of a certain culture are harder workers, we hire them. If we believe our spouse does not truly love us, we close our hearts. Our beliefs inform us over time, giving us guidance about how to behave. This is beneficial from an evolutionary perspective because it makes for faster responses to stimuli and quicker reactions to the external environment. Each new event does not have to be reinterpreted, as there is already a sense of how to respond. We already know what to do. We have, for example, learned a great deal about how to act in a given situation, or with certain people, by virtue of their gender or race or age or social status. We treat the cop, the waitress, grandma, grandpa, and street people differently. Different social roles create different social relationships. Our beliefs about those social roles help maintain predictable interactions and thus promote greater social order. This allows for economy in our information processing. Beliefs are highly informative yet compact. They are socially efficient and this gives them great value to humans.

> In essence, our beliefs provide prepackaged information. They remind us of how we feel about things and shade our sense of the way things should be.

Although such a system provides a basis for greater efficiency in processing life experiences, it is not without a cost. The problem is that not all of our beliefs will be beneficial to our success and progress. Some of them may be quite limiting, and their influence can overshadow an entire life journey. Do such limiting beliefs transform or heal as we get older? Unfortunately, that is not necessarily the case. Just look at the older people around you, and you will unfortunately see significant depression, anger, resentment, and fear. I had one client who came in to do hypnotherapy for the first time when she was in her eighties. She had been taught something about herself as a child that was very limiting, and some seventy-plus years later she was finally ready to work on it. She was an inspiration to me, that it is never too late to begin healing. She was also an excellent example that age alone does not cure our problems. Over time the problems can actually worsen as life circumstances reinforce and strengthen limiting beliefs. Limiting beliefs can potentially self-correct if good fortune provides highly supportive and healing environments. The best strategy, however, is not to wait passively for things to change, but rather to consciously work on removing limiting beliefs and replacing them with empowering new ones. Life is too precious and too short to wait for the good times; there is no excuse big enough or good enough. The time to find peace and success, to be our fullest, happiest self is right now.

The Good News

Research in developmental and cognitive-social psychology shows us that beliefs are constructed over time through our interactions with the world. Beliefs are, in essence, built by hand; they are not part of our original landscape. As with any type of fabricated structure, our belief constructs can be well-designed or poorly designed. Well-designed beliefs provide a foundation for greater enrichment for ourselves and ultimately for the lives of others that we touch. Poorly designed or dysfunctional beliefs, on the other hand, can impose extreme constraints on our quest for success and happiness. Because our beliefs are learned, not etched in stone, in principal they can be intentionally modified through new learning.

So why not just reduce the limiting beliefs and increase the facilitative ones? What prevents that? It is not necessarily a simple or direct process, as the self's belief system is designed to be somewhat stable. This stability is useful for two reasons. First, beliefs, as predefined mental constructs, give us a consistent sense of self and place, providing a degree of psychic stability in our lives. Second, beliefs allow humans to interact with each other and the world around them in predictable and efficient ways. These two qualities help us to function in the social and natural world. We know who we are, what we believe, how we feel, and how to act. We can also predict the behaviors of other people to a reasonable extent. All of this helps to reduce the amount of unique information we must attend to and deal with. The price of that relative stability, however, is the challenge in transforming beliefs. If we want to work with beliefs constructively, we need to be able to attend to various stabilizing phenomena that may include limited awareness, denial and false logic, selective attention, avoidance, and inertia.

Limited Awareness

The first task is to become aware of our limiting beliefs and recognize what we need to work on. Why is that an issue? No doubt we are all conscious of many of our beliefs. They can be expressed readily. "I believe that the candidate I am voting for has the best solutions to the nation's problems." "I believe that we are destroying the earth." "I believe that black, brown, red, white, and yellow people are lazy, slow, greedy, dirty, addicts." "I will die for my faith. I believe in you, Almighty Ahura Mazda, Allah, Aphrodite, Belenus, Buddha, Buku, Chac, Danu, Gluskap, Jehova, Jesus, Krishna, Kuan Yin, Mercury, Thor, Vulcan, Zeus . . ."

There is no problem reciting many of our numerous core beliefs. Even when we voice them, however, we do not recognize them to be beliefs. They are concepts that we have held for so long, or that are so widely ascribed to by our society and social groups, that we do not even think to question them. Such beliefs are no longer seen as ideas; they are understood as our truth.

> Cultural beliefs are held as truth by virtue of their encompassing nature, possessing immense reach across time and space.

Two major sources of such unconscious beliefs are culture and family. Cultural beliefs are held as truth by virtue of their encompassing nature, possessing immense reach across time and space. Cultural beliefs about race, age, gender, sexuality, intelligence, good and evil, health and healing, work, and all the rest of it can be profoundly limiting for humanity. Religious, political, social, and economic beliefs have bloodied and oppressed people since the beginning of civilization. The Italian astronomer, Galileo, was denounced by the Inquisition and had to recant the Copernican notion of a planetary system with the sun at its center since it conflicted with the beliefs of the church. Ignaz Semmelweis, a physician practicing in Vienna in the 1800s, went mad trying to educate doctors to wash their hands between procedures. These doctors believed it was acceptable to do an autopsy on a cadaver and then proceed directly to delivering a baby. The great spiritual activist, Mahatma Ghandi, was assassinated because of his belief in nonviolent activism. As we are all inextricably woven into our culture, and it into us, these cultural beliefs become part of our fabric, part of our core self system. They can be very hard to see as limiting ideas, and if seen, perhaps even harder to resist given the forceful currents of a predominant world view around us.

The second type of invisible belief comes from the microculture of the family. These are our core beliefs about self that were planted before we can remember. They come from our more immediate social world, first from parents and family members, then from friends and close community. The parent who tells the child that he or she is chubby, tall, awkward, skinny, shy, dumb, lazy, or in the way, will reinforce a self-concept oriented around those attributes. That information becomes core self-knowledge, a piece of the individual's essential sense of self.

Such powerful and pervasive social influences root beliefs deeply. As such our awareness of them can be quite limited at first. Movement away from the ignorance of limiting beliefs requires that we begin to look for and recognize such beliefs. Our healing begins with self-awareness, with making invisible influences more visible.

Denial and False Logic

After limited awareness come the unconscious cloaking mechanisms of denial and false logic. I have all too often listened to clients who will not acknowledge an obvious life problem or who eloquently espouse logical reasons for their destructive behaviors. They are almost convincing. It is truly sad to listen to someone defending a behavior that is clearly self-destructive. How well we hide those inner demons behind the curtain of denial, protecting them like precious lovers. How effectively we justify their value in our lives. We are addicted to those relationships. We are intoxicated for a while, so we do not want to stop and look at what we are doing. We have been taught over the years to self-destruct. So we fulfill the manifesto of self-limitation written for us so many years ago by emotionally crippled parents and guardians or by our wounded cultures. If we are to be free, it is absolutely essential that the spell be broken.

Our beliefs are not gospel. They are not universal truths. They are artifacts of specific times, places, and influential people. They may in fact be quite untrue, like the swan thinking it was an ugly duckling. It was not a duck at all, but it was trapped in that duck belief until contrary evidence provided new insight. The challenge with beliefs, however, is that we want to believe them, so we unconsciously devise rationales and world views to support our beliefs, even when those beliefs hurt us and those around us. We create a framework of false logic to hold them all together. Since this is not real logic, but a self-serving logic, anything can be rationalized. This makes breakthroughs more challenging. Reality testing is not done, and the status quo is maintained, potentially forever. To exit such a potentially endless self-cloaking loop, we need a method that can make this denial and false logic system more permeable to allow in contradictory information. What we need is a method that creates a space where we can honestly and openly explore our dreams and visions.

Selective Attention

Another important cognitive process protects against the introduction of new empowering beliefs—selective attention. This is a process in which the focus of our attention is narrowed. If we are looking for quarters in our coin jar, we will have selective attention for the large, silver-colored objects. All other items will take a secondary role in terms of our attention and awareness. This same process of selective attention plays a key role in belief maintenance. The world is pure stimuli—sights, sounds, feel, smell, and taste. There is too much information coming in for the brain to process, organize, and make meaning of it all. One of the strategies our brain uses to deal with all of that input is to just pay attention to the most pertinent fragments of the data stream. As an example, a fish swimming in a pond spends a good part of its day looking for food. The fish, however, does not jump at just anything floating by. It has a food construct, an internal representation of what bugs on the water surface look like. This food information helps the fish to selectively attend to certain types of stimuli. The fish sees an object

> The world is pure stimuli—sights, sounds, feel, smell, and taste. There is too much information coming in for the brain to process, organize, and make meaning of it all.

that is about the right size, shape, and color, and it responds. That is why fishing lures work. Our belief constructs allow us to do the same thing. They assist us in filtering life data, allowing for quick matches against a large array of experiences, helping us to know how to respond to things.

Selective attention is a valuable cognitive process that helps us to deal with the vast quantities of life information constantly flowing in through our senses. It helps us focus our awareness and make decisions. This function becomes problematic, however, when we selectively attend to things that support our limiting beliefs. If we believe a child is bad, we will notice the bad things the child does more than the good things. A critical boss will rarely notice the good efforts of employees, but will almost always notice their mistakes. If someone believes that he or she is incompetent, that person will notice their failures and overlook their successes. In life we selectively attend to the things that fit our beliefs, and we avoid or downplay the things that do not. If we want to facilitate our transformation, we need to temporarily deactivate this process so we can allow in new information that is outside our normal range of tolerance.

Avoidance

A phenomenon somewhat related to selective attention is avoidance. Selective attention is more of an internal process while avoidance is more external and behavioral. They produce similar results. A person with strong religious or political beliefs will not actively seek out contrary information, and if encountered such information is often discounted or refuted. We often avoid things, places, and other people that do not support our dominant beliefs. Conversely, we actively pursue things that do support our basic beliefs. We do not want to disrupt our belief homeostasis with contradicting information. We prefer experiences that perpetuate our core conceptions of self and others. Birds of a feather flock together, constructs seek matching constructs, and people with shared beliefs, cultures, and world views associate with each other. This is natural to some extent due to the ease afforded by shared beliefs, the bond of common culture and perceptions. Shared beliefs are familiar, comfortable, and predictable. For healing and growth to occur, however, it is useful to experience new realities, outside our norms of behavior and knowledge, ideally in a safe and controllable context. Personally, some of my greatest learning has come when a wiser person gave me an idea that was the exact opposite of what I had always believed.

Inertia

Once we rise above limited awareness, denial, and the other protective mechanisms, we must then confront the reality of inertia (or the inertia of reality). Transformation may require working on beliefs that have roots deep in our psyche. I remember one summer helping out a group of people who were starting a meditation center up in the mountains. In an effort to build community, it was decided that all the initial work would be done by hand with no machinery. There was a very old, very large tree stump in an area where a retaining wall was going to be built. We had to dig it out. The more we dug, the more roots we found. It took many days and lots of sweat, but we did finally remove that stump. We had a vision of the end state, the clear space; we had the intention to get there; we persisted; and it happened. Anyone embarking on the hero's journey of belief transformation faces a similar challenge. The surface symptoms may belie the expansive psychic structures below. There may be deep roots to contend with. Success takes patience and persistence.

Why are these roots at times so deep? Through a lifetime every person gets some powerful messages. The parent who is impossible to please conveys a message to the child that no matter how much effort is made it will never be enough. That child will have to work and work to prove her worth. The alcoholic parent who never comes through with promises, is not there for birthdays, or your recital, or your ballgame, instills the belief that people are not reliable and not to be trusted. The parent who sexually, physically, or emotionally abuses, teaches the child that the world is unpredictable, cruel, and unsafe. The family that is authoritarian, noncommunicative, and punishing teaches the child that showing affection or speaking one's mind is inappropriate and dangerous. The family that discourages exploration, crushes ambitions, and discounts dreams teaches the child to settle for less. These experiences build up in the child's psyche, like layers of sedimentation becoming encrusted, heavy, and thick. The child takes in each experience, sees it, hears it, feels it, remembers it, day after day, week after week, year after year. The five-year-old child has over twenty thousand possible waking hours of contact with parents, community, and culture. A twenty thousand–hour lesson in one's competence, attractiveness, worthiness, gender, race, and social class is a very, very big lesson. It is huge.

All of those beliefs, shaped by family and culture over generations, come to represent a substantial psychic mass that does not stir easily. There will be resistance to starting transformation (limited awareness and denial) and inertia once the process begins. Such beliefs persist in the mind and body as memory, as expected response, as personal and group history. They are deeply rooted in the heart of each person's self-identity and within that person's family and culture. They become part of the basic fabric, the basic understandings of our life. Challenging and changing such beliefs will require persistent and committed effort, but it is definitely possible. It is definitely possible for us all to heal, grow, and learn new things. We all have the potential for true success as humans. It is part of who we are.

Self-Fulfilling Prophecy

The various belief-sustaining processes, such as denial, avoidance, and selective attention, help us to maintain our self-identity. They help us to maintain a consistent and congruent self. They help us to have, in a very fundamental sense, a human social existence. Since our beliefs are so important to our functioning in the world, they are protected by our psyche as if a guard were at the door preventing strangers, in the form of new information, from entering. Only information that is acceptable to the current ruling paradigm is granted access. In this way our beliefs sustain a reality. They become self-fulfilling. Every belief we hold predisposes us to sort reality in favor of that belief, and that affects how we will think, feel, and act. Our beliefs help to maintain a life that remains consistent with existing beliefs, or expectations for better or for worse. What we believe shapes the activities, people, and places that we interact and identify with, and that reinforces our thoughts, behaviors, and life choices. If we believe deeply that we are marginal or incapable, it will dramatically affect our choices in life. We will lead a life that matches those beliefs. If we believe we are capable and strong, that will similarly shape and direct our life in profound ways. We will make choices that foster growth and success. We will associate with people and places that support and empower us. Ultimately our belief system is a truly powerful selecting, directing, and self-maintaining energy with the power to drag us down or take us higher.

So the challenge is clear. Each of us deserves to have liberating visions, to be free to move toward our greatest dreams, and to be radically alive. To do that, we must first heal our limiting beliefs by transforming or removing them. They need to be replaced with empowering beliefs that can carry us to our desired future. The trick is getting past the guards, working through the resistance of very deeply rooted old beliefs, and laying the foundation for empowered new beliefs within the core architecture of the soma and psyche. Fortunately for us there is a very effective way to do just that.

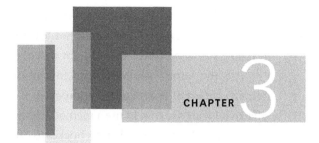

mind-body learning

All humans learn and adapt. From the moment we are born, we learn about ourselves, others, and the world. In addition to the obvious things we learned in school, such as reading and writing, mathematical concepts, painting or singing, we also learned many subtle things about our place in the world. Family and culture all significantly shaped our self-concept, what we believed ourselves to be. Those beliefs, both limiting and liberating, are learned concepts. Fortunately, because they are learned there is also the potential to unlearn them if they do not serve us well. The question is not can we change our beliefs, but rather, how can we change them.

Approaches to Learning

The process of transforming beliefs is a learning process, and human beings have a natural talent for that process. It is part of our essential human nature. How do we approach this unique task of learning new beliefs and transforming old ones? There are certainly many ways to learn, from classroom to private tutorials, from books to active participation. Each method has a proper time and place. For example, learning calculus is a very different task than learning to snowboard. Calculus is a cognitive skill, while snowboarding is more of a motor skill. Those two activities require different methods of instruction for effective understanding and successful application. One would not teach calculus in the same way as teaching snowboarding. It would not make sense.

It is the same with belief transformation. Teaching different tasks requires different instructional approaches if we hope to be efficient and effective. Ideally we should use a method that best fits the task to be learned. We use an ax to chop wood and a bucket to carry water. The method must suit the task. In selecting the best method we must first consider both the task and the intended result. What will the person be able to do differently at the end of the journey? Learning is about a person progressing along a path to a destination. When that person arrives at the designated point, he or she will be different. That person will have more capacity to solve problems, perform physical tasks, and to understand others. The keys to success on the journey are: getting clear on the destination and picking the best path to get there.

Relearning Beliefs

If our goal or destination is transformation of belief, then the path or learning method must be appropriate for achieving that end. Whatever method we choose must effectively deal with the self-protective nature of our beliefs. Beliefs are resistant to change by virtue of a variety of internal protective mechanisms. If we hope to have any success with deep belief transformation, then we need to select a path or method that can take us to our destination of new beliefs, successfully navigating through those protective mechanisms. Changing beliefs is not like memorizing phone numbers. Many of our most obstructive beliefs are hidden from us. They abide deep within the architecture of our soma and psyche. They are ingrained neural and biochemical patterns that are vested with powerful emotions and thoughts. If we want to succeed in this transformational journey we must absolutely understand and creatively work with these aspects of our human nature.

When we think of learning, most of us probably recall our school days. Certainly that type of learning was productive for many societal purposes, but perhaps it is not well-suited to the job of belief transformation and empowerment. Why not? Western education serves the needs of modern society. Those needs reflect movement over the past several centuries toward a culture increasingly oriented to industry, science, and technology. Mass migrations from the land and farms toward cities and factories were movements away from seasonal and spatially based realities to more immediate time-based experiences. This movement from nature to technology spurred the need for new models of education. The move to industrialize mandated a more literate, technically educated workforce. In response, western society developed efficient systems of public education to meet those specific needs. The new educational systems were not designed with the intention of cultivating personal enlightenment or self-understanding. They were based on the need for productive workers, the needs of a materially oriented culture.

Many of our most obstructive beliefs are hidden from us. They abide deep within the architecture of our soma and psyche. They are ingrained neural and biochemical patterns that are vested with powerful emotions and thoughts.

The western approach to imparting new knowledge is very linear. It flows sequentially through predetermined developmental stages, first the ABCs, then recognizing and writing simple words, then reading books, and so on. Western learning is highly verbal, including both the written and spoken word. It also places a significant emphasis on analytical thought, emphasizing logic and reason. The preponderance of content taught in such schooling is cognitive, mainly facts and ideas. This type of education helps to support and maintain a material-oriented society. But it is not necessarily the appropriate strategy for deep personal transformation. Personal growth is not the intended purpose of the dominant Western educational paradigm. For learning paradigms that emphasize the goals of deeper personal insight and transformation, one place we can look to is the East. There in the forests, monasteries, and ancient texts, we find a wealth of methods designed specifically for the journey of inner transformation.

Mysticism and Metamorphosis

The modern Western cultures and ancient Eastern cultures developed different yet somewhat complementary approaches to transforming the individual. The modern West emphasizes learning based on language, logical analysis, and linear development of understanding. The ancient East, by contrast, employed methods for deep transformation that relied more on imagery, intuition, and holistic understanding. Interestingly, these complementary styles from the West and East are represented in the two hemispheres of our brain. Seminal work done by researchers such as Roger Sperry, who received the Nobel Prize in Medicine in 1981 for his contributions in neuroscience, helped reveal the brain's hemispheric laterality. His pioneering work showed that each half of the brain has unique qualities. In a general sense, the left hemisphere is more predominantly involved with language, logic, and the known. That half of our brain would be like Western culture—the rational side. The right half of our brain, on the other hand, is more associated with intuition, imagery, and the unknown. That hemisphere would be the East—the ineffable, mysterious side.

Both halves of our brain are involved in developing and maintaining our belief constructs. The left hemisphere of the brain, however, the side of language, logic, and what exists, plays a larger role in maintaining certain aspects of the self within society. Sir John Eccles, a Nobel Laureate in physiology, has described the left hemisphere of the brain as the source of civilization because it possesses our verbal capacity. That capacity allows for internal dialogue helpful in remembering our role and place, approval and disapproval, what shames and excites. Here we find the words to describe self to self, the words that describe us to others and others to us. The logic functions of this hemisphere can help to maintain our belief integrity or continuity, creating the rationalizations necessary for preserving beliefs in the face of contradicting information. The left hemisphere also influences our perception of what is, of self as object, which can support our sense of personal history and of transhistorical continuity, the sense of self over time. Interestingly, it was many years after researchers understood the functions of the left brain before they grasped the role of the brain's right hemisphere. The functions of the right brain were not as evident, being aspects of another cultural paradigm. Researchers could more readily see and document the Western-oriented functions of the left hemisphere of the brain than those of the Eastern-oriented right brain.

The Eastern Perspective

If it is true that the left hemisphere more actively maintains the social self and its belief system defenses through language, logic, and linear thought, then it would be beneficial to have a learning state or method that circumvented that hemisphere to some extent. Ironically, much of Western psychotherapy is verbal and logical, more analytical, more of the left brain. This is in keeping with Western education and culture. Although a very valuable approach, we can see how this method potentially approaches the self head on, diving face first into the tsunami. This is not to criticize such an approach, as talking is profoundly important for insight and change, and indeed many psychotherapists use a variety of nonverbal methods. However, if the left brain's penchant for logic and language is fundamental to belief maintenance, then it would be productive to seek another path for transformational learning. Einstein once said that one cannot solve a problem at the level of the problem.

To apply that idea here, we would ideally not approach the self at its own maintenance level. That is like letting the opponent get first pick of weapons. That match will not be favorable to us. We will be fighting against their strong suit. Perhaps that is why in the East, the issue of self-transformation has been approached in a very different fashion. Their approaches are more right brained. Eastern approaches to self-transformation commonly involve a general reduction in system activity, an inner quieting. There is a reduced reliance on logic and language and a greater use of intuition (such as insight through deep meditation) and feeling (such as veneration of the chosen deity or path). Also, these systems do not typically employ logic as a principle path to self-transformation. The Eastern methods place a premium on reducing internal dialogue, on quieting down the body and mind. In their efforts to find the existential self, they silence the worldly self, the socially constructed belief self, and its self-preservation mechanisms.

The Age of Hypnosis

The world is changing. Now in the West we are hearing a voice calling for the mystical, for things Eastern, for knowledge that is more intuitive, visceral, and personal or perhaps universal. Since the 1960s there has been a continual growth in the integration of ancient Eastern concepts and methods in our culture. I began my own spiritual journey many years ago, dropping out of college for a while to become a meditation and yoga teacher. I too was looking for approaches to inner growth and transformation, and I found them in those ancient teachings. There are Eastern approaches to learning, thousands of years old, that serve those needs. There are also contemporary Western methods similarly suitable to this unique type of transformation, such as biofeedback, autogenic training, and hypnosis.

Transformational methods such as these from both the East and West may prove to be especially appropriate for the task of learning new beliefs, employing methods that reduce system arousal, reduce reliance on logic and words, and open pathways for the introduction of empowering new information and understanding. Of these approaches hypnosis is an ideal learning strategy for belief transformation. It is a highly flexible self-help resource that produces an extremely effective learning state for working on issues of mind, body, heart, and spirit. It is a profoundly useful tool that we are just beginning to truly recognize and understand in the West, with many distinct advantages for transforming core beliefs.

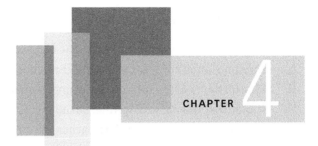

CHAPTER 4

the hypnotic advantage

Self-hypnosis is one of the best methods for belief transformation. It is an advantageous tool for transformation for several reasons. It encourages goal clarity, focuses attention, quiets any inner resistance, and facilitates new learning in a way that is almost effortless.

Clarifying Goals

Learning is a journey. It is about a person moving down a path toward a destination. Effective learning requires that we have some sense of our destination, of a goal. One of the great benefits of regular self-hypnosis practice is that it encourages us to work with and clarify our goals. Through this regular goal-setting process, we begin to increase our awareness of the possible, reduce our denial of what is wrong, and admit to ourselves what we truly want. The process of goal clarification will be examined in greater detail in chapter 6.

Focusing Attention

Hypnosis employees techniques that focus attention. Learning requires attention, a state of readiness, a mind and body receptive to receiving new information. No attention, no learning. Simple. Do you remember grade school? A room full of fidgeting, talkative children is not a very productive place for learning to occur. The teacher needs to get the students' attention, to have each child present in body, mind and spirit. Self-hypnosis does that. Self-hypnosis initiates the process of effective learning by focusing our attention. This is accomplished through body centering and other methods that begin to shift attention toward a more internalized, quiet state. It is very much like shaking a rattle to distract a crying baby. Once you have the baby's total attention, the infant often will not only stop crying but even begin to smile. Focusing shifts the infant's state of awareness. In such moments of concentrated awareness the world is fresh, our worries cease, and we are open to receive what is coming next. We are ready to learn in that moment.

Reducing Resistance

Hypnosis reduces our innate resistance to change. In the last chapter the concept of brain laterality was introduced. As you recall the left hemisphere of the brain is more engaged in language and logic. The right hemisphere of the brain is more involved in imagery and intuition. In addition to the unique role that each hemisphere plays, the brain's overall bioelectrical activity also has important effects on our consciousness. This activity can be measured as brain waves via an electroencephalograph (EEG). An EEG charts the peaks and troughs of a brain's electrical activity. One can look at these brain waves and determine how active or quiet a brain is and where the activity is located. Both the area of activity and the amount of activity affect our perceptions and the nature of our moment-to-moment consciousness.

During the twenty-four hours of a day, our brain exhibits four major bioelectrical states. Each of these four states is characterized by unique brain wave frequencies, measured in cycles per second, and designated by the Greek letters delta, theta, alpha, and beta. Delta, the slowest frequency waves, reflect activity in the range of one to three cycles per second. Delta waves predominate during deep sleep. These slow waves indicate a reduced level of mind-body activity. At the other end of the spectrum are beta waves. Beta activity is measured at thirteen to thirty cycles per second. Beta waves are normally observed during periods of increased mental and physical arousal. The other two brain wave states are alpha, which is a slower eight to twelve cycles per second, and theta, at about four to seven cycles per second. Alpha waves are associated with quiet alertness; theta activity with dreamlike reverie.

Increasing Beta Alpha and Theta Brain Waves

Increased alpha and theta brain waves are commonly observed during relaxation, meditation, and hypnosis. The various elements of a hypnosis session help to reduce arousal, lowering the brain's beta level activity. Beta waves occur when the brain is engaged in daily activity. They reflect a continuum of arousal. Simple activities like doing laundry or buying groceries will probably be in the lower beta range. Someone experiencing a traumatic event, such as a near car crash, will probably be in a very high beta state. The beta brain will be more active, potentially associated with more internal dialogue, while engaged in noticing, analyzing, and commenting. It can be a very busy mind and that busy mind can affect our peace and happiness. If you close your eyes and count your thoughts for a minute and then multiply that by the hours of waking activity, you will see that there are potentially thousands of thoughts a day. Many of those thoughts reinforce our existing limiting belief constructs. They are like an army of stone masons on patrol ready with bricks and mortar to fill in any breach in the vast wall of our beliefs, like a psyche's immune system, fighting off foreign ideas.

As the beta state begins to quiet we enter alpha. The alpha state is productive for learning because alpha is alert, yet quiet. It begins to take us below the noise of the beta brain's engaged voices. It is awake and receptive, an excellent quality for assimilation. As we move down through the alpha state into theta, we access yet another productive space for learning. We still find an awake mind, but it is now moving into a more dreamlike

> When we quiet our thoughts we can begin to disengage the aspect of the self that is built on inner dialogue, on the words that define self and others.

state. The theta state is a place of reverie, the daydream mind, the generator of spontaneous imagery. Very young children, about age three or four, spend more time proportionally in the theta state than adults do because of their level of brain development. That accounts for some of their play behavior with imaginary friends. They are in a very real sense living in an imaginary world at times. Theta is a very deep yet conscious state. It is a place where we can still hold intention, still do the work, but encounter much less resistance. Theta activity is observed in adults in the hypnagogic state between waking and sleeping, in deep hypnotic states, during daydreams, in fantasy and creative thinking, and during meditation and imagery.

When we quiet our thoughts we can begin to disengage the aspect of the self that is built on inner dialogue, on the words that define self and others. This strategy is in keeping with the ancient wisdom of Eastern meditation practices where the meditator seeks to quiet thoughts in order to better see into reality and understand truth. Such inner quiet is a return to innocence, a return to the Garden where we can be reborn. In self-hypnosis we also seek this quieting of mind and body to facilitate deeper learning. It is like slowly crossing a river to get across to the other side. Once slowed we do not have to worry about being knocked down and carried away. The crossing is easy, even enjoyable and refreshing. Somehow, almost magically, the river is parted and we find ourselves on the other side.

Thinking Holistically

In addition to creating helpful changes in brain-wave activity, hypnosis also facilitates hemispheric changes useful to processing transformation. As inner quieting deepens, the left hemisphere of the brain, which is normally the predominant of the two hemispheres, begins to relinquish its hold. The right hemisphere of the brain is given a greater voice in the cocreation of awareness. As right hemisphere dominance increases, the various functions of the left hemisphere, such as selective attention, become less active. The protective functions are being turned off. The guards are falling asleep. The mind and body are now accepting new ideas without checking each one for personal identification. Other left hemisphere processes, such as the emphasis on verbal language and logical processing, can similarly decrease. As the right hemisphere comes into play, the activities of imagery and intuition are awakened. Our problem-solving process becomes more global, more insightful, more dreamlike. We are now using both halves of our brain more fully, and due to reduced dominance of the left hemisphere, we reduce resistance to novel input.

Learning Vicariously

Another value of self-hypnosis is the potential to experience a world of possibilities. The deeper hypnotic state is a very creative dreamlike space. As we move into this dreamlike realm, we access an increasing capacity to tolerate ambiguity. Dreams are made of inconsistent images and concepts and illogical associations, yet they are readily accepted while dreaming. The dreaming mind is very comfortable with illogical premises and foreign ideas. In a dream you can fly your bicycle to an English garden to have a conversation with a long-departed loved one. It all seems quite plausible, quite natural. In the hypnotic state the mind can similarly consider all types of possibilities that would not be believable to the conscious mind because of learned limits. Such tolerance allows for the introduction of new conceptions of self, potentially inconsistent with long-held beliefs. In the hypnotic state we can experience ourselves winning the race, giving the best talk of our life, being in a wonderful marriage to a loving person. It all becomes believable.

This aspect of hypnosis provides an opportunity to learn through vicarious experience. As the state deepens and the imagery becomes more absorbing we can have very real encounters. In those moments we are actually in the imagery, we are part of it, not separate. We are there. At that level the information is real. Just as in a dream, if we are being chased by a tiger, we awaken feeling frightened with a pounding heart. It is a very real experience at that level, and we learn from the experience, just as we would in an active waking state. The new information is now in our mind and body. It has left its desired mark. In this way we can learn from such indirect or vicarious experiences and use this learning to profoundly affect our beliefs.

Introducing New Information

Another major advantage of a self-hypnosis strategy is its effectiveness in introducing new information. Methods such as meditation and biofeedback are wonderful for helping to cultivate the receptive mind-body state useful for deep transformation. However, they do not specifically introduce new transformative ideas. New information is often a key step in learning. New information can help correct mistaken ideas and behaviors. A golf pro, for example, might teach someone a better way to hold the club. That bit of corrective information can completely transforms the amateur's game. With the introduction of even a small piece of appropriate information, it is often possible to achieve dramatic personal improvements. Such learning can occur in self-hypnosis through the introduction of suggestions into the receptive learning field of a quieter, more creative mind-body space.

Producing Change Effortlessly

Self-hypnosis is able to transform us without struggle. This is very important given the magnitude or mass of some of our beliefs and their consequent inertia. We need a user-friendly method (accessible, flexible, and effective) to work on old static beliefs. A belief developed over many years will probably take some time and commitment to unravel. Fortunately self-hypnosis is easy to use anywhere and at any time. In self-hypnosis we plant a seed in the fertile soil of the receptive mind. In this nonlinear, creative field of mind-body energy, our dream begins to grow. With sufficient practice (as in any learning process) a new belief structure begins to take form. At some point, when a critical mass is reached, new thoughts, abilities, and behaviors emerge. We do our inner work and then without really trying to change, something shifts at a deep level, and we are different. We feel different, we act differently, we are different. Once the new belief locks in, our perception and experience of life changes, right before our eyes.

It is not uncommon in working with clients to have them come back a week later completely unaware that a change has already occurred. When asked about the presenting issue, they will have to reflect on their week to realize that their issue has not been a problem. The change can be that effortless and natural. I was once working with an executive who bit her nails. She was very successful and was quite embarrassed about this behavior. We did two sessions. At the second session she came in and talked about several things, never mentioning her nails. So I inquired about the nail biting. She reflected for a moment, looked at her lengthening nails, and said that she had not chewed on them at all that week. Then she said, "I wonder whether hypnosis had anything to do with it?" Well, after twenty years of nail biting without any change, I think so. Given the subtle nature of hypnotic transformation, however, it is not surprising that people act this way. In the linear, conscious Western orientation to learning, we are used to applying effort to make things happen. In hypnosis the magic just happens, just as the seed becomes the plant once it enters the proper soil. We plant the proper suggestion deep into the creative hypnotic mind-body energy field and transformation occurs. Learning occurs at a core level. Fundamental changes in beliefs about self, others, and the world become reality.

Once the new belief locks in, our perception and experience of life changes, right before our eyes.

a one-minute method

If you are like me, you do not want to read an entire book to find out how to do something. You want to start using a new skill now. This book is full of principles, techniques, and applications that will help you to become quite skillful in working with self-hypnosis over time. For those of you eager to begin now, however, the essence of all of those skills can be condensed to this simple formula:

- Induce and deepen a quietly focused mind-body learning state.

- Send transformative suggestions to that deep mind-body state.

- Come back refreshed and ready for life at a new level.

So, for those of you in a hurry, here is a one-minute method to get things started.

1. Sit or lie comfortably.

2. Close your eyes.

3. Take three deep breaths and release all tension.

4. Do the following:

   - Imagine you are holding a two-inch energy ball in your hand.

   - Squeeze it, physically squeeze it.

   - Pretend that the harder you squeeze the more it resists, that your forces match equally; you cannot modify the shape of the ball.

   - Tell yourself, "The harder I squeeze, the deeper I go inside."

   - Continue to squeeze for a minute; then absolutely, totally, completely release everything.

- Feel yourself dropping down deep inside.

- Give yourself your suggestion, "I feel incredibly energetic, confident, strong, loving, or . . ."

- See the desired outcome; see a future image of that outcome.

- Feel the positive feelings associated with that outcome.

- After a few minutes, tell yourself that you are, "Coming back feeling refreshed, relaxed, and ready for an amazing day."

- Then slowly open your eyes.

That's it. Now here we go!

PART TWO

the **elements** of
SELF-HYPNOSIS

CHAPTER 5

preparing for self-hypnosis

The process of self-hypnosis as outlined in this book follows a simple five-step path. These steps are: visioning, focusing, deepening, transforming, and concluding. Each step will be described in detail in the following chapters in a modular fashion. The final section of the book will tell you how to integrate these elements or modules for use with a wide variety of issues, including finding relationships, making more money, improving health, achieving greater success in sports or a career, feeling more confidence, enhancing inner peace, and much more. Like most important life journeys this process requires that we take time to prepare to get the most benefit out of the effort that we put in. A little preparation can often make the difference between success and failure. Everyone has taken exams and knows that studying generally improves the outcome. Study time supports success. Similarly, before you sit down to do your own self-hypnosis, you will want to prepare for the journey. This chapter provides some specific ideas about how to optimize the practice of self-hypnosis to increase your effective use of this tool and your ultimate personal success.

Right Attitude

One of the keys to making life work is to have the right attitude. It is the same with self-hypnosis. If we approach this task with positive expectation, and take patient, persistent action, our deepest dreams will come in time. It all begins with the right attitude.

A NATURAL EXPERIENCE

Self-hypnosis helps us access a state of mind and body that is ideal for transformative learning. This is a natural state that we actually go in and out of all the time. For example, everyone daydreams at times. Everyone has experienced reading a book or watching a movie and becoming completely engrossed in the story, oblivious to the outer world. If we overhear a conversation of someone talking about grandparents, our mind slips into a memory of our own grandparents, momentarily absorbing us into the past. During those times the mind does not go away, it just shifts to a more internal place, less distracted by the outer world. That is the mind we use in self-hypnosis. It is part of our nature, something we experience so transparently all day long that we do not really notice the shifts in and out. If we can shift to this state while watching a movie or reading a book, then we can learn to do it any time. This is something for which we all possess a natural capacity; it is something we can all learn.

DEPTH OF THE HYPNOTIC STATE

Some people believe that hypnosis produces a state of complete oblivion, a total loss of awareness of everything that is going on. That is probably where people's fear of loss of control comes from when they think of hypnosis. In reality, however, there are many levels of consciousness that individuals experience in hypnosis, some more superficial and some deeper. Generally, in a very deep hypnotic state an individual will not be aware of their external environment, as their mental focus will be very internal. In a lighter hypnotic state, though, the external environment remains in our awareness. The important thing to remember is that the goal of hypnosis is not the subjective experience, but rather the outcome of the process, what happens afterward. My observations over the years have shown me that people can have both surface and deeply internal experiences and that both states produce positive results. The results are what matters, and I have not necessarily found the depth of the hypnotic state to be the determining factor in this regard.

POSITIVE EXPECTATIONS

Self-hypnosis is powerful, so the more you allow it to work, and expect it to work, the better. Positive expectancy will help support the process and increase your success. Imagine the following situation. Two seven-year-olds are playing in their first piano recitals. One child has a supportive parent who always encourages her to do her best. The other child has a parent who always expects her daughter to fail. Which child will perform better at that recital and enjoy the process more? Life is more pleasant and productive when our loved ones support our success. The same can be said for encouraging and believing in ourselves. Be positive and expect the best from your practice.

PATIENCE AND PERSISTENCE

Successful self-hypnotic transformation requires two qualities: patience and persistence. Change is a process. People who want everything to improve or to be different overnight, without any commitment or effort on their part, are going to be frustrated souls. It is important to be patient with your process. Persistence is equally imformant. One of the simple reasons that many people do not succeed in life is that they lack persistence. They give up too early. The sad thing is that they may be well on their way when they give up, like the guy in the joke who swam halfway to Hawaii then turned around because it was too far. Bunker Hunt, one of the world's wealthiest people, once said, "To be successful, you must decide exactly what you want to accomplish, then resolve to pay the price to get it." Have a clear vision, put in the work, and persist until it is done. Hypnosis is very powerful, but it will not change our lives overnight. Most things take time. If we are patient and persistent with our dreams, using self-hypnosis to empower them, they will come.

TAKING ACTION

Self-hypnosis is not a magical process. If your hypnotic suggestions are to make more money, that goal will probably not manifest as the sweepstakes patrol coming to your door. It is more likely that those suggestions will activate your creative inner mind, bringing you ideas about what steps to take next, helping you feel strong enough to follow your dreams, making you more confident about your skills, and providing greater clarity about what your unique gift is. Very often self-hypnosis changes lives by empowering people to take action, moving them toward their dreams more confidently.

BEING GRATEFUL

It might sound funny that gratitude could improve success, but it can. Gratitude is essentially a state of appreciation for what we have. If we express gratitude for the little changes as they happen, we build enthusiasm for our growing success. If we refuse to be satisfied until we have the mansion then our negative mind state will slow our progress. The ultimate outcomes may look different than we expect them to. If we are not grateful for the little changes we accomplish, we may completely miss the fact that our answers are coming through now, because we will be looking for something else. Through our practice, results will come, at the perfect time and in the perfect way. There is an inner wisdom at work here so the answers may look different than what our conscious mind expects or wants. Appreciate success in any form, big or small; it is all progress. Gratitude in its own right is a very powerful healing attitude. If we all had more gratitude for life's simple pleasures, the world would be a much better place. How do you think your life would change if you were more grateful?

Right Context

One of the nice things about self-hypnosis is that it does not require special circumstances—no special garb or postures, no special context. You can do it almost anywhere and at any time. Once you have the skill you can drop into your hypnotic work space in short order. It becomes easy to mix it into the events of your day as needed.

SESSION LENGTH

One of the nicest things about hypnosis is that it does not take much time. All you really need is a few minutes, literally, to do some quick work.

It is a quick, anytime, anywhere process. You can easily do a number of brief sessions throughout the day as needed. You can do microsessions right before an event, such as a sport performance or an exam. Actually, several short sessions during the day are probably better for self-hypnosis than one long session, since it may be harder to find the time to do a long session. Just a few minutes of practice now and then will begin to set a new pattern in motion. Of course if you have the time, you can do a twenty-minute session or even longer, but mini-sessions are excellent.

IDEAL CONDITIONS

It is possible to do self-hypnosis almost anywhere since you are working inside a self-generated mind-body space, a virtual environment if you will. Yet despite this flexibility it is desirable to have an appropriate setting when possible. Ideally you will use a quiet and calm location. Peaceful music can enhance the process. Music can help create a secondary source of distraction, absorption, or emotional evocation. Well-chosen music can help elicit a specific emotional tone that is useful for channeling your work in different directions; the tone may be quiet or it might be expansive or powerful. As a general rule, however, it is useful to select quieting and relaxing music, as calmness supports the hypnotic process. Turning down the lights will help reduce sensory input also. Put pets outside the room. They will be attracted to your quietness and will want to sit on your lap, which will be distracting. If you have children or a partner, tell them you need a few minutes of quiet time and close the door. It is better to not do hypnosis right after a meal as the blood is shunted to digestion and alertness decreases, making the mind and body less alert. You could fall asleep and self-hypnosis is not a sleep state. Similarly, doing self-hypnosis late at night can be challenging as tiredness may produce sleep.

LESS-THAN-IDEAL CONDITIONS

Those are some ideas for creating an ideal environment for self-hypnosis. If, however, you find yourself doing your self-hypnotic practice at the office, on the road, or in the million other less-than-perfect places of life, then at least try to find a quiet out-of-the-way corner if possible. Close your eyes when you do your inner work. Self-hypnosis can be completely invisible to others. No one will know what you are doing. It will look like you are resting for a few minutes, when in reality you have an entire change process occurring within. When I fly I often do several hours of inner work. To those around me it looks like I am asleep. This is very helpful if you do not feel like talking to anyone. Because self-hypnosis is not context dependent, you can do it whenever you need it, wherever you are. When I find my mental wheels spinning, accomplishing little, I take a five-minute self-hypnosis break to focus my mind and get back on track. That is usually sufficient to get things rolling again.

Right Understanding

Before we proceed to the specific techniques of self-hypnosis, it would be helpful to present a quick overview of the five-step model we will be learning. Each element of this process will be explained in detail in the upcoming chapters:

- **Visioning**—select goals and prepare for the session (*chapter 6*)

- **Focusing**—induce the hypnotic state of consciousness (*chapter 7*)

- **Deepening**—use methods to deepen the hypnotic state (*chapter 8*)

- **Transforming**—give self-transformational suggestions (*chapter 9*)

- **Concluding**—complete the process and return to activity (*chapter 10*)

VISIONING

It is important to select appropriate value-based goals to prepare for your hypnotic session. Determine what you want, your desired goal or outcome, what needs to be transformed.

FOCUSING

Induction methods take our attention from the external to the internal, from the diffuse to the focused. These methods withdraw our awareness from the outer world, helping to quiet our mind and body. A number of induction methods useful for focusing attention and going into the hypnotic learning state quickly and easily will be introduced in chapter 8.

DEEPENING

Once the hypnotic mind is engaged you will want to deepen that state. If we were to describe the induction process as entering a house, then deepening would be like proceeding into the house to explore other rooms. There are many methods for deepening that we will examine in chapter 9, including relaxation, imagery, hypnotic phenomena, and direct suggestion.

TRANSFORMING

With the deep mind activated we are more responsive to new transformative suggestions. Hypnotic suggestion is a fundamental element in this process. These suggestions are like the rain that washes away old residue and creates new streams. Those drops of rain ultimately become a mighty river heading to the sea.

CONCLUDING

At this point the hypnotic work is done, the suggestions have been given. This final step offers an opportunity to provide final suggestions, to create expectations for even more effective future sessions, to deepen the effect of the current session, and to come back prepared for a great day (or evening).

Other Forms of Help

Every job requires the right tools. You would not paint a house with a hammer. You could do it, but it would be very slow and inefficient. Self-hypnosis is not a replacement for professional treatment. Someone with a serious problem, whether it is physical, emotional, social, or spiritual, will benefit from professional attention. A potential limitation of self-treatment involves not seeing the actual problem or the best solution. You cannot see your own face without a mirror to reflect it back. We are often the last to really understand our own issues, in part due to the self-protective nature of the habitual mind. Also, symptoms can be misleading. I knew a woman once who had persistent headaches. She thought she had sinus problems. When she finally consulted her doctor, he was suspicious of the symptoms and sent her for scans. It turned out she had a very serious brain tumor. That was a year after the headaches started. The point is that in our lives we need both self-care and professional care. There is a time and place for both. Working with a skilled professional can often help remedy a problem quickly and more completely. If professional care does indeed turn out to be the best strategy for you, self-hypnosis may be a great adjunctive treatment. Be open to receiving the help you need from others, be it doctor, clergy, or coach, in addition to healing yourself. Why suffer needlessly. Life is short enough. Be happy.

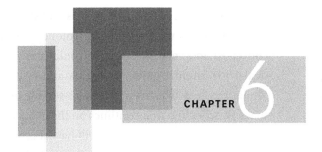

creating clear goals
—*visioning*

There are many benefits to having a clear vision that add tremendous value to life. One definite advantage of a strong vision is that it concentrates our actions. By having a sense of where we are going, we automatically limit alternatives and channel our efforts in a specific direction. Clarifying goals is the beginning of powerful action.

Committing to a Path

Developing a clear vision narrows our range of options and allows us to commit to a path, a plan of action. This makes for a more effective life, and examples of this are evident in all spheres of human endeavor. When contractors build a house they start with a blueprint of the finished structure.

They would never just buy materials and start building things randomly. That would be a waste of time and money, resulting in something poorly conceived and very unsound. It would ultimately require extra effort to deal with unanticipated problems and issues as the project evolved. Similarly, when an artist is painting a still life or a portrait she initially will make sketches and draw outlines on the blank canvas. An excellent athlete will have a game strategy. Successful businesses are built on solid business plans. Any serious endeavor in life deserves a thorough plan to efficiently and effectively reach the desired goal. Realistic plans may evolve over time to accommodate new information and changing circumstances, but the core vision remains intact, providing the foundation for powerful action.

> It is always our choice, to scatter our precious life energy carelessly or to apply it for the highest good.

The implications of clear vision are actually profound if we consider the precious value of our life. No one knows how long life will last. It is all too often that we hear the unfortunate news of some young person who has died unexpectedly from an illness or in an accident. I have known several younger people who unexpectedly died: one from a drug overdose, another in a violent crime at work, and one from a sudden heart attack while jogging. Death came without warning, and I suspect none of them were truly prepared. While we are alive we have time and life energy at our disposal. They are ours to use as we see fit. Like a gift of money, some people will use these resources wisely and others will squander them. It is always our choice, to scatter our precious life energy carelessly or to apply it for the highest good.

One very prudent use of time is to achieve greater clarity of vision. Focusing our vision creates a natural parsimony in living. It helps us to receive the most benefit for the least effort. There are so many possibilities in life and never enough time to do all of the things we might hope to do. If we have a clear vision, however, our priorities become obvious, and consequently we know how to use our time and where to direct our life force. So the effort we apply to developing and clarifying our vision will in turn save us time and energy as we pursue our highest dreams. A clear vision will reduce false starts, random movements here and there. Every step becomes purposeful, powerful, and productive. A clear vision is truly a key to successful living.

Empowering Action

A second profound benefit of a clear vision is that it empowers action. If a person's hair is on fire there will be a powerful commitment to finding water. Such clarity of need concentrates our energy, our intention, and our effort. If we took several handfuls of small pebbles and tossed them in the air, they would fall with little force, but if we put them all in one cloth sack and threw them, the same stones would make a great impact. Concentrated energy is powerful. A laser, for example, takes regular light, focuses and organizes the light particles, then shoots them out as a powerful beam. A laser starts with regular light particles, like those from a table lamp. Such light is disorganized, incoherent. A laser takes light particles and makes them coherent and organized. That order creates power. In a similar way, a personal vision makes our ideas and actions more organized, focused, and coherent, and that increases our potential to do powerful things. We have time for so many things, but few people take the time for the critical task of refining their life vision.

Getting Feedback

A third significant benefit of having a clear vision is that it creates a meaningful framework for feedback, which is essential for efficient learning to occur. Life continually offers us feedback. Having a vision or goal encourages us to use that feedback to determine whether or not we have made progress. It is like taking a trip to New York from California. We will recognize our progress as we pass signs for Wyoming, Nebraska, Iowa, and Pennsylvania. Since we know our destination, the signs along the way provide evidence of the correctness of our path or process. If we noticed signs for British Columbia or Mexico, we would see that we were off course. Without a clear picture of our final destination, life's feedback becomes less helpful, less meaningful. A clear vision makes all feedback more relevant and obvious.

Building Enthusiasm

Finally, a clear vision builds excitement and enthusiasm. It helps us to paint a clearer picture of the future we want. If we do not see the future in our mind, if we do not feel it in our heart, then it is harder to generate the requisite enthusiasm we will need to move through life's inevitable obstacles. We need a vision to overcome the inertia that comes from fear, our limiting beliefs, and old habits. Because our vision is set in the future, it gives us something to move toward. If this beacon is brilliant enough it will draw us forward from darkness into light. That brilliant vision awakens us to be the leader of our own lives. Commitment to a vision is a strong statement to oneself and the world. It says, "I deserve to have a dream. I deserve to be happy. I deserve to be free. I deserve to live my life. I deserve to be here. There is something that needs to be done. I have something to offer this world."

Start with Values

For a goal to be truly powerful it should be built on a foundation of your life values. If goals do not have a value-based foundation, they may actually be counterproductive. For example, if you have a goal that runs against a deep personal value then you will probably encounter unconscious resistance to progress on that goal. The student who is in an engineering program to please parents but would rather be a writer may be a very frustrated soul. Part of that person's energy may obstruct progress because their goal is other-based, not coming from self. Such goals will cut against one's deeper personal sense of meaning. To the extent that our goals match our values, there will be real passion and energy behind them. Look at each of your goals. Look at what it will bring you, its highest benefit. Then see whether it matches your key values.

Consider Where the Issue Resides

In addition to values and goals it is helpful to know where a problem, challenge, or issue resides. This requires some differential diagnosis. Why diagnose the problem at all? Because if we do not know what is broken, we will not know what to fix. When mechanics work on cars they do an initial diagnosis to determine whether the problem is electrical, mechanical, or just being out of fuel. Without that step their work would be less efficient.

The form of personal assessment used in this book does not focus on causal roots from the past. Unraveling such threads can be a very complex task. The approach taken here for self-hypnosis considers the layer that is most active in relation to an issue. Think of life as a sphere with three layers. At the center of the sphere is the person. The second layer is their behavior. The outer layer is their environment. So the entire sphere consists of three dynamically interacting elements: the person, their behaviors, and the environment the person interacts with. One of these layers may be the most useful for intervention with a particular problem. There is also the element of time to consider—one's past, present, and future. More on that in a moment.

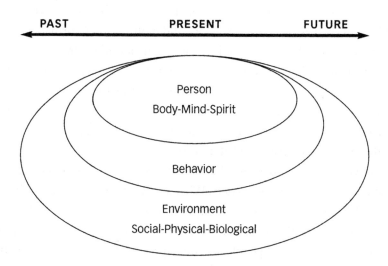

PERSON FACTORS

The person includes everything that happens inside—thoughts, feelings, internal body states or physiology, sensory processes, ego experience (the sense of I), and spirit. For example, I have worked with clients on weight management issues in my practice. One woman I helped had spent much of her adult life going from one diet to another. Like many people she attributed her weight issue to eating the wrong foods, in the wrong amounts, at the wrong time. All her solutions, however, were only temporarily successful. Like most dieters she would chronically gain the weight back despite her best efforts. After our conversations it became apparent that she was eating in part to appease emotional needs, feelings of emotional pain, sadness, and loss—aspects of the person layer. We did some hypnotic work at that level, including specific suggestions of eating healthy, low calorie foods and exercising. During the ensuing months, without much effort, she lost about thirty pounds. More importantly, she has become a happier, more integrated person. Weight lost much of its significance as her life came into a more natural balance.

BEHAVIOR FACTORS

The behavioral layer is what we do, the things others can observe or notice about us. It can include habitual or addictive behaviors, interpersonal skills and challenges, verbal behaviors, and motor skills. A former client of mine had been seeing a psychologist for many months. The psychologist had been analyzing her relationship with her father as a possible cause of her high anxiety. She came to my office for acupuncture for another issue and happened to mention her anxiety. In my interview I asked her, being the brilliant fellow that I am, if she drank coffee. She did, over a gallon of caffeinated coffee a day. So what do you think I suggested? I advised her to cut down to eight cups a day. The next week she came in and told me that she was feeling much less anxiety. What a surprise. So here she was being treated for anxiety with the assumption that it was psychological. I was amazed that her therapist had never asked her about coffee, but psychotherapists are mind people, not body people. We always see the world through the filter of our professional training. Her problem was not an emotional one, it was a coffee drinking habit, a behavior. We got her to cut down on coffee—change a behavior—and her anxiety improved dramatically. She stopped her therapy.

ENVIRONMENT FACTORS

The outer layer of our life is the environment, which includes social, physical, and biological factors. I once had a client with chronic low back pain. He was receiving medical attention to no avail. He came to me for hypnosis. Interestingly his symptoms only appeared when he was having difficulties in his marriage. My assessment was that this was his unconscious mind's way of telling him to heal his home life. He had been in a lot of denial about his marital difficulties, wanting to believe he had a happy family. His body, however, was trying to tell him to pay attention to this issue, a social environment issue, before it got worse. I reframed the issue, did some work on having healthy relationships, and got both member's of the couple into counseling together. Their relationship and his back problem both improved. Interestingly, the only time his back acts up now is when they are off balance, which provides him with useful information that he can use to stay more conscious about the healthiness of his social environment. That is body brilliance.

> Self-hypnosis . . . is generally not as focused on the past as some therapies are. It is more solution oriented, focused on the present and the future. It emphasizes where we are now and where we want to be.

Look Forward

The interplay of person, behavior, and environment all move through time and space. We have a past, a present, and a future. Self-hypnosis, however, is generally not as focused on the past as some therapies are. It is more solution oriented, focused on the present and the future. It emphasizes where we are now and where we want to be. That is one of the things I love so much about this healing method. You do not have to know why you have your challenges. You mainly just have to be aware of where you want to end up, your vision or goal, what kind of life you want to have. Certain types of hypnotherapies do deal more with the past, such as exploring the traumatic incidents of childhood. If that is what you really want or need to do, that is beyond the scope of this book. You would be best served doing that type of work with a licensed psychotherapist who does hypnosis. It is very important to have someone qualified to guide that process in the event the material that surfaces is disturbing. Be prudent.

The Process of Visioning

It can be helpful to determine whether a problem is something inside our person, like a troublesome thought or emotion, whether it is a habitual behavior, such as lighting a cigarette every time we talk on the phone, or whether it is about our environment, perhaps a need to change some social relationship. If we can determine the correct layer of the challenge, we can be more specific in our strategy for dealing with it. So take a little time to consider where you have been (if that is pertinent), where you are now, and most important, where you want to be. Remember not to be too concerned about the problem or obstacle. The emphasis is on what you want. Focus on the outcome, your desired or preferred goal. The mind-body learning state of self-hypnosis will find a path to your destination. It is like an internal compass, always finding north. Get as clear as possible about the goal you want, and if possible be specific as to whether you are working on transforming thoughts, feelings, physiology, behaviors, environments, or a combination of them. Develop a clear goal and then prepare to enter the transformational space of self-hypnosis.

Visioning Activities

Spending some time now to determine or refine your goals and visions is a key to success in the remainder of this book. The following exercises are designed to help you awaken a clear and powerful vision. Take a while to work through each exercise. Even if your goals are already clear to you, this process will be a valuable opportunity to refine them and recommit to them even more deeply. This is a very important part of the process. Every minute spent here will reward you with more truly abundant success in your future. Do yourself a favor and take time for your vision now. It will be of benefit to the rest of your life.

PERSONAL VALUES LIST
Time: Five to ten minutes
Materials: Pen and paper

For this exercise, focus on your values. Dreams that are built on things we value deeply possess more power. Everyone has a set of core life values.

Those values reflect what is most important to us. You might value family, or freedom, or health, or compassion, or excellence. If we base our visions on deep personal life values, those visions will propel us forward in amazing ways.

Exercise

Take five or ten minutes and write down your responses to the statement: "I value . . ." Do not edit, do not organize, just write. Get down to the bare bones of what is important to you. Do not stop. Write down whatever comes to mind. "I value health, good food, nature, fast cars, a house in the country, world peace, travel . . ." When the time is up, go through your list and pick your top three values and circle them. Once you have selected your top three, pick the most important value from that short list. On a separate sheet of paper, write these values down, top value first and then the next two, and keep the list where you can see it occasionally.

Prioritize and List Your Top Three Values

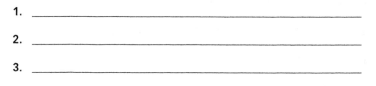

1. _____

2. _____

3. _____

108 FUN THINGS TO DO

Time: One hour
Materials: One long sheet of paper and a pen

Having fun is liberating. It opens us up, unties us, sets us free to explore with no holds barred. Letting yourself have fun and dream is a good way to start stretching your mind. It helps create the proper perspective required to bring an exciting future into focus. If we never play, if we never dream about the possible, then we limit our capacity to reach new heights. This next exercise is a great way to play with dreams, to get into the habit of dreaming about what you want.

Exercise

This exercise could take an hour or more to do, so set aside some time. On a sheet of paper list the 108 things that you want to do in the next ten years, or in your lifetime. In ancient India 108 is a magic number. Do not put down things that are impossible or unattainable. Do not list "fly to the moon" if that is highly improbable or "become president" if you do not really mean it. By contrast do not limit yourself to things that are practical or customary for you. Dream bigger. If you have always wanted to live in Paris for a while, then by all means put that on your list. This is a long-term perspective. List whatever you want to do. Absolutely and positively include all the fun things you want to do in your life—sky dive, surf, help build a temple, do a fund-raising bike ride for a good organization. This is a mind-expanding list. Be sure to have fun with it. Date your list and keep it around. One person I know put her list on her bathroom door as a daily reminder. She is having fun checking off her items one by one.

People who do this exercise tell me how amazed they are when they start checking off items and seeing how many of those things they are now doing. It is very empowering to see the fulfillment of dreams, especially expansive dreams. So take some time and do the list. It does not have to be 108 items, but head in that direction. Put down as many items as you can think of, and add to your list over time.

Three of Your Most Fun and/or Motivating Goals

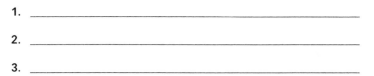

1. _____

2. _____

3. _____

FUTURE VISION

Time: One hour
Materials: Pen and paper

Having a vision of the future, a rewarding and successful future, is very compelling. When it is clear and strong it inspires us. There is an excitement about that future, a desire to become that vision. Such a vision awakens our motivation to take action, to overcome obstacles, and to move forward. A clear, compelling future vision is a treasure map that can lead us to gold.

Exercise

Write a success story on what your life will be like six months from today. Write it as if it were a diary page from a day in the future. For example, let us say that today is actually July 30. I would write, "It is December 30. I am sitting on my couch thinking about what an amazing year it has been. I have been working out five days a week and feel better than ever. I can now do twice as many sit-ups as I could six months ago. I am spending much more time with my love ones, including that great camping trip we did in the mountains. Work is better than ever. I got the promotion I was going for and my new work environment is fantastic . . ."

Since this is a short-term vision, for six months, you will want to make it practical. Include the key things that you want to have accomplished in six months and write them down. Make them observable, measurable things. Writing down items like, "I will feel better" or "I am making more money" is much too abstract. You need to make this real, so be specific, with tangible items that are accountable: "I ran a ten-minute mile," or "I brought in three new accounts." Also, make them likely enough that you can get behind them, get excited about them, make them happen. This is a vision you are going to commit to. Put the achievement date at the top of your paper, and then mark your calendar for that date. Look at the items in your imaginary diary page periodically and use regular self-hypnosis and affirmation to help you meet your specific objectives. This is another great way to get a sense of the things you are willing to work toward.

Three Major Future Accomplishments, Date

1. _____

2. _____

3. _____

Not Sure of Your Vision

If you have done some of the exercises and are still not sure what you want, that is fine. Even if you truly do not have a clue, you are not alone. Many people are working on getting a clear vision about what to do in various aspects of their lives, such as career, relationship, or where to live. Self-hypnosis can be a very useful method for finding a clear vision. If you lack vision regarding your career path, for example, then you can use hypnosis to help you find the right career. Then you can use self-hypnosis to help obtain the perfect job. Using hypnosis this way will probably be faster than just sitting and waiting for something to occur to you. Self-hypnosis is a way to tap into our creative wisdom and to more accurately understand our deepest dreams and desires.

The actual method for reaching greater goal clarity is quite simple. First do the One-Minute Method of self-hypnosis described on page 28. For your suggestion try something like, "I am totally clear on my purpose and my goal. I know exactly what I want to do. I am confident and powerful and taking active steps to achieve my dream. I am totally clear about . . ." Specify what you are clear about—the type of work you want, where you should live, what you should eat. See yourself looking happy. See yourself knowing the answer to your most nagging question. Also, remember a time in your life when you were completely clear about something and then bring that feeling memory into your session. Perhaps you once bought a great car. You were absolutely clear that it was the one, and indeed it was. Remember that moment you bought it and let yourself have that "This is the one!" feeling again. Once you have accessed that feeling, tell yourself that you are clear on your current goal—who to marry, where to work, what career to pursue, whatever you are seeking to clarify. This will imprint that clear-minded feeling from the past onto your current issue. It truly helps. So let that confident mind-body feeling empower your self-hypnosis statement. Do this for several weeks and see what happens.

Still No Vision

Over the years I have found that one of the best steps to take for attaining clear goals is to cultivate and deepen self-love and self-confidence. These two qualities provide the basis for knowing who we are and what we are capable of. Most of us probably have a few limiting beliefs tucked away inside somewhere. Inner doubts can overshadow our shining vision, obstructing our path to success. We need to deal with these doubts. Doing self-hypnosis for greater self-love and self-confidence begins to remove the dust and withered vines from our vision window. We must not be afraid to love ourselves, to feel our power, to be who we were born to be. We all have something to offer the world, and that gift comes through our commitment to living an honest and powerful life.

Ultimately, if we do not get answers it can mean several things: wrong question, wrong timeframe, complex questions that have no simple answers. If it is the wrong question then we will never get the right answer. If we keep getting nothing meaningful back then it may be useful to look at our value base again to see whether our desired vision truly reflects our deeper truth. If we do not really want to move to another city, and our question is about where to move, then it will not be surprising if we get no answer. The question in that case is not where to move to, but rather, whether to move. Be honest with yourself when asking your questions. Follow your highest truth. The answer can also avoid us because it is not our time to know yet. A first year college student may eagerly inquire about what work he or she will be doing in twenty years. In reality that can be a hard thing to know as career-related aptitudes, interests, and skills may not be fully expressed or recognized yet. That unfolding is partly a process of time and experience, a process of living. If this is the reason answers are not coming, then you can ask questions relevant to earlier stages of the issue, and work on those pieces first. In this way the answers and insights will build sequentially to a fuller understanding of the big vision. Finally, some questions are so complex that there is no simple or single answer. In such a case breaking the question down into components may be useful. In the end if the answers are not forthcoming for any reason then do not waste time fretting. Just consider your current reality as perfect for now. Live in the present with passion and conviction, knowing that your passion is ultimately moving you deeper toward your destiny.

Be open to the magic of life, to synchronicity, gifts from on high, and grace. Things may not come in the form we requested since what we desire is not always in our highest good. Learn to notice and appreciate the cascading gifts as they come in. Do not be afraid to receive the gifts life is giving you. Also, do not be resentful when the gifts do not seem to be enough. Learn to accept all of life graciously and be patient and persistent as your vision refines over time. Learn to love what you have, and then in time you will have what you love.

> Learn to accept all of life graciously and be patient and persistent as your vision refines over time.

Practice Notes

Jot down your experience and insights from trying different visioning activities. What worked best for you?

_____

_____

_____

_____

_____

_____

_____

_____

_____

_____

_____

_____

_____

_____

_____

_____

_____

_____

_____

_____

_____

_____

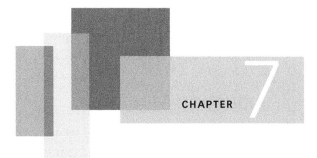

centering attention—
focusing

The hypnotic state we use for transforming beliefs is different from normal waking consciousness, so it must be accessed or induced. Giving yourself suggestions in hypnosis is not like giving yourself a suggestion in normal waking consciousness. In hypnosis we introduce verbal suggestions and images to a deeper inner space, which then works with that material to construct new possibilities. For hypnosis to do its work, we need to access that special learning place.

The induction methods we are about to examine provide an entry point for self-hypnosis practice. Induction methods are specific techniques that take us from the outside to the inside, from conscious mind to inner mind. The induction process is like coming home, entering our house and standing in the vestibule. We have entered the house and are no longer outside, but we have not yet begun to move deeply into the structure to examine its various living spaces. The induction process is the transitional area that we migrate through when moving from conscious mind to deep mind.

Induction Methods

The essence of induction is the focusing and narrowing of attention. Induction methods help the mind to transition from the active outer consciousness to a quieter, more internal state. Depending on the method employed, transition can occur gradually or very abruptly. Although there are many different types of inductions, all of them work by essentially disengaging the conscious linear mind, temporarily slowing down the normal thought processes and focusing mental awareness. This puts the body and mind in a better state to receive suggestions to facilitate the transformation process.

Have you ever noticed that a loud, sudden noise can cause your breath to briefly stop, your mind to quiet, and your awareness to orient toward the sound? The state may only last for a few seconds while the sound is being analyzed, but in that time the mind and body are still and focused. That shift from normal mind to a quiet, focused mind is an induction into a new state, a state ready for responding and learning.

Induction methods employ a variety of approaches to elicit a similar centering effect. They include creating an inner focus, using repetitive stimuli to entrain the mind, attention fixation, creating mental imagery, employing hypnotic phenomena, and making direct suggestions. Descriptions of these primary techniques are presented below with sample techniques. Experiment with them and notice how each induction method feels. At the end of the following section you will find four induction exercises with more detail to give you a set of specific approaches to use. Try them and see what works best for you.

INNER FOCUS

Inner focus, as the name implies, is the process of directing your attention inward, as in meditation. In ancient India preparatory methods known as Pratyahara were used prior to meditation. These methods helped withdraw the mind from the sense channels, turning the focus inside.

Technique

Lie down comfortably and scan your body slowly, noticing how your body feels. Tell yourself mentally that you are lying down, that you feel your legs, your arms, your head on its cushion. Describe to yourself in some detail what you feel, such as pulsing, twitching, vibration, warmth. Focus on pleasant rather than unpleasant sensations. Focus your mind in the moment. To a large extent that is what the hypnotic induction methods do. When the mind begins to focus on some aspect of the body, such as breathing, physical position, or muscle relaxation, there is a shift away from the distractions of the outer world toward a more narrowly focused inner world. This focusing helps prepare the mind and body for hypnosis. Practicing a body scanning process can be very centering.

REPETITIVE STIMULI

Have you ever been mesmerized listening to the sound of ocean waves or a gentle spring rain? Perhaps nine months in the womb listening to the muffled sound of a beating heart trains the mind to find comfort in rhythm. Not surprisingly numerous induction methods employ the repetition of monotonous, rhythmical, sensory stimuli for fixing our attention. An example of this is the repetitive visual pattern of a swinging watch or pendulum.

One pleasant and very effective method is to use some type of instrumental music. There is quite a bit of nice ambient music around these days, new age or space music, which is perfect for this type of work. It is not totally monotonic, but it does have a soothing, often rhythmical nature. The music should be relaxing and soothing. Some of the environmental sound pieces work very well in this regard also, such as the sounds of ocean waves or rain, as they provide the natural auditory patterns we love and that may remind us of rich images we have experienced, such as a walk in the forest or watching a summer thunderstorm move over the desert.

Technique

Sit or lay down comfortably. Use something from your environment that has a repetitive visual pattern, such as a moving clock pendulum. Or use auditory stimuli of your choice. Allow yourself to watch or hear the pattern you have selected and notice how your body and mind feel as they become entrained to the pattern.

ATTENTION FIXATION

In this approach you will focus on some object to fixate your attention. Just like a honeybee is enamored with a flower and its nectar, if the mind is engaged in something attractive the normal stream of thought begins to slow down creating the potential for entering a more focused inner space.

One ancient Indian Pratyahara method is a technique called *tratak*. In *tratak* you gaze steadily at an object, such as a candle flame. The reduced visual input, if you can actually keep your gaze relatively still, has the effect of quieting the mind. You can also gaze at a mountain or the ocean, a tree, a framed picture of some natural scene, or a geometric pattern (like a Tibetan *thangka* painting, a mandala), a crystal, a small shining object, or any other pleasant stimuli. All of these methods gently hold the mind's attention allowing it to become quiet and restful.

Technique

While sitting comfortably, pay attention to specific body spaces, such as the space between your eyebrows or your heart region. Just feel the energy there. It is subtle but present if you quietly pay attention. Feel the area as tingling energy or a ball of warm light.

MENTAL IMAGERY AND ABSORPTION

This induction method uses the mind's ability to generate absorbing images. It is like daydreaming. When the mind is engaged in a daydream, we lose track of the world around us and become open to new ideas and inner experiences.

Technique

Think of a beautiful place that you have actually been to that you find particularly comforting, relaxing, and safe, such as a mountain meadow or the ocean. It may be a real place or a favorite science fiction or fantasy environment. Choose any image you like, as long as it is safe and relaxing. As you begin to picture the scene, you will automatically be drawn into the imagery. Let yourself go into that place. Let yourself see the colors, hear the sounds, and experience the sensory nature of it. Let yourself feel the relaxation and comfort of that place.

HYPNOTIC PHENOMENA

Hypnotic phenomena will be explained in more detail in chapter 8. For the moment, however, we can say that such phenomena are both ways into and effects of hypnosis.

Technique

Catalepsy (paralysis) is one of the more common hypnotic phenomena used for induction. In catalepsy a body part is made immovable temporarily, such as having the hands stick together. For this practice bring your hands together and interlace your fingers. Press your hands together. Tell yourself that the more your hands stick together, the deeper inside you go. Tell yourself that they are completely stuck and that you are deep inside. Then try to pull them apart. If you are good at this particular phenomenon you will not be able to pull them apart until you tell yourself that you are unlocking them and they are returning to normal.

DIRECT SUGGESTION

You can enter the hypnotic state by telling your mind that you are going inside into a deep quiet inner space. Direct suggestion can be very productive. Often all we need to do is to give ourselves some direction or suggestion, and the desired result will follow. This is a helpful practice to use with any of the other induction methods you choose. Whichever one you employ, it is generally useful to tell yourself that you are going deeper and deeper inside, moving toward a very powerful, wise, and creative place within yourself—into a place of comfort.

Technique

Sit quietly with your eyes closed. Notice how your body feels. Tell yourself mentally that you feel wonderful, that your body feels very relaxed, quiet, and calm. Do this for several minutes, then sit quietly and notice how your body feels. You should feel more relaxed and quiet. Now tell yourself slowly, calmly, and repetitively that you are going deeper into relaxation and peace. Repeat this for a few minutes. Stop and notice your feelings.

Am I in a Hypnotic State Yet?

There are a variety of hypnotic symptoms or indicators that provide evidence that the mind and body are entering a different state. These can be subtle or obvious, and they will vary from session to session. They can include small twitching movements as the muscles respond to inner images and relaxation, reduced heart rate and breathing, greater muscle relaxation, slower responses to stimuli, warmer hands and feet, stomach sounds as the body begins to relax and encourage improved digestive function, and increased responsiveness to suggestion.

Accept Experiences as They Come

An accepting state of mind is very helpful for transformational practices. Allow everything you experience during your sessions to be perfect just the way it is. There are going to be noises in the environment, carpenters hammering, buses going by, people talking. If you consider those noises to be bad, thinking they are an annoyance, then they will indeed be a deterrent. The best thing to do is to incorporate them into your experience by telling your mind that these sounds will help you go deeper. Try it. It really helps. Use the same approach for anything that would be potentially distracting. Tell your mind that everything you feel, hear, smell, think, or imagine, on any level, is just going to help you go deeper into a wonderful state of relaxation and peace. There are no distractions, only deepening experiences.

Use pleasant experiences to assist you too. Perhaps you are doing your practice outside and you feel the warmth of the sun on your skin. You may have some wonderful, relaxing music playing, or you can smell the flowers on your table. Allow these pleasant sensations to awaken your gratitude. A grateful mind is very quiet and spacious because it is content.

Trust Your Process

The hypnotic experience will undoubtedly vary from session to session because the mind and body are always changing. Some sessions will be faster and deeper than others. You can imagine how frustration with such variability could be counterproductive to a state of inner focus and peace. You cannot have both, inner peace and frustration. Trust your process. One of the wonderful ironies of hypnosis is that you cannot try harder to do better. In hypnosis the harder you try, the less you get. It is in letting go that the magic occurs. It is like the words of St. Francis, in giving we receive and in dying we are born. When I work with clients I sometimes have to tell overachieving individuals to let the process happen. Their trying to help gets in the way of their outcome. Perhaps it is a good lesson for our Western minds that, at least with hypnosis, entering the hypnotic state emphasizes being more than doing.

Induction Exercises

Here are a few specific induction exercises explained in detail for you to explore. Experiment with them and choose one or two to work with for now.

LOOK UP, HOLD, DROP DOWN

This is a simple and effective exercise that I often teach clients for their home self-hypnosis practice. There are three steps to the process—inhale and look up, close eyes and hold breath, release and drop down. You can do it sitting or lying down. To begin, just look straight ahead with a relaxed gaze. You can look at something peaceful, such as a blank wall or out the window at a tree or the sky. Keep your head still; you will be moving your eyes, not your head. Inhale. As you inhale, slowly look up, as if looking at your eyebrows. Once the inhale is complete, continue looking up, and close the eyelids. Hold your breath for a count of ten. Keep the eyelids closed and the gaze upward. When you reach ten, exhale quickly, letting your gaze quickly drop back to the starting position. Totally release your muscles on the exhale and imagine that your body is dropping down. The sensation is like gently dropping through your chair into a vast open space. It is very pleasant. Then slowly open your eyelids partially, and repeat the process two or three more times. Each time, open your eyelids a bit less. On the finale exhale keep your eyelids closed and continue to relax deeply.

FUSED EYELIDS

Sit comfortably and gaze at some object, such as a picture or a blank wall. Tell yourself that your eyelids are getting very, very heavy. Keep gazing and telling yourself that your eyelids are very heavy, that they want to close. Soon your eyelids will feel heavy and will close. Next you begin to suggest catalepsy. Repeat to yourself that your eyelids are so heavy that they will not be able to open. Use phrases like, "My eyelids are so incredibly and comfortably heavy." This increases the incentive for the eyes to close and stay closed. Tell yourself that as your eyes close and become fixed together, you will go deeper and deeper inside, into an incredible place of healing and creativity. Keep repeating the phrase, allowing your eyes to become heavier and heavier until they close shut. Tell yourself that they are incredibly heavy, locked shut, wonderfully, comfortably heavy, so heavy you could not open them even if you wanted to. Try to open them, try hard if you want. Tell yourself that the more you try to open them the more locked they become, taking you deeper and deeper inside. They will not open until you are ready to open them. You can test this if you want. If you are good at this method your eyelids will not open until you tell them that they can open. Be aware of your locked eyelids and allow yourself to go deeper into the feeling. Sit until you are ready to come out. When you are ready, tell yourself that your eyelids are releasing and that they feel perfect. Then come out ready to see a whole new world of possibilities.

MAGNETIC HANDS

This excercise is done sitting up. Pleasant music is a nice accompaniment to the process. Close your eyes. Hold your hands about sixteen inches apart. Your forearms should be several inches above your lap, parallel with your lap. Your palms should face each other. Tell your hands that they will be drawn toward each other as if two magnets were pulling them together. Tell yourself that as your hands move closer, you go deeper and deeper into a wonderful transformational state. Your hands will move toward each other. Let your hands continue to move together until your palms are close or touching. Let your fingers interlace and then tell your hands that they are melting together. Let them become one energy, feel them dissolving together into one energy. When you are ready, tell your hands to slowly separate and float down toward your lap. Tell your hands that they will feel great, better than normal. Let them sink down and rest. Come out feeling refreshed and relaxed. Notice how you feel, the warmth of your hands, the energy in your body, anything else you are aware of. Enjoy it.

HEAVY HAND

In this method your hand is going to become very heavy. Close your eyes. Take your left hand (engages the right hemisphere of the brain more, possibly useful for self-hypnosis) and place it on your lap if you are sitting, or on your abdomen if you are reclining. Lift it up about three inches. Tell yourself that your hand is getting heavier and heavier. Tell your hand that it is going to sink down toward the body. Let it move by itself. Keep giving your hand the suggestion that it is getting heavier and heavier, wanting to sink down. Tell yourself that as your hand sinks down you will go deeper and deeper into a peaceful inner space. This is very important. You want to let your mind and body make the association between the event (such as the heavy hand) and going deeper inside. Let the hand sink down to the body. As it rests on the body tell yourself that the heaviness of the hand will take you even deeper inside. Let the hand continue to become heavy. Tell yourself repeatedly that the hand is getting heavier and heavier with each breath out, immovable. Let it become incredibly heavy, immovably heavy. Keep repeating to yourself that as it becomes heavier you go deeper and deeper into your place of healing, vision, and power. Suggest to yourself that your entire left side is becoming very heavy and relaxed. The heaviness of the hand is spreading throughout the entire left side of your body. Continue these suggestions until you are ready to come back. When you are done you can tell your hand and your body that they feel normal, better than ever, very relaxed and refreshed.

Practice Notes

Jot down experiences and insights from trying the various methods. What worked best for you?

_____

_____

_____

_____

_____

_____

_____

_____

_____

_____

_____

_____

_____

_____

_____

_____

_____

_____

_____

_____

_____

_____

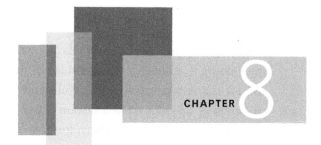

quieting mind and body—*deepening*

Visioning

Focusing

Deepening

Transforming

Concluding

In the previous chapter, hypnotic induction was compared to coming home and entering your house, stepping over the threshold. Continuing that analogy, the deepening component of self-hypnosis is like taking off your coat and shoes and settling into a comfortable chair by the fire to relax. First we enter by focusing (induction), then we deepen the state for greater creative potential (deepening). In this chapter we will examine a variety of effective methods for that deepening process. Special consideration will be given to relaxation as a deepening method because of the unique therapeutic value it provides. Other deepening techniques we will explore include direct suggestion, counting down, imagery, and hypnotic phenomena.

Relaxation

People typically find hypnosis very relaxing, which is one of the reasons they enjoy doing it. Although relaxation is not necessary for a deep state to occur it is a very common and useful element. One reason we focus on relaxation as a basic part of a session is that it is therapeutic in its own right. Relaxation therapy has been found to help ease muscular tension, headaches, neck and back pain, high blood pressure, mild phobias, insomnia, and depression. It is safe, effective, and easy to learn. Although relaxation alone is therapeutic, it is even more productive when combined with hypnosis. Adding imagery and hypnotic suggestion significantly increases the transformational focus of the process and consequently produces much more powerful effects.

Relaxation Techniques

Try the following relaxation techniques, then use them as part of your self-hypnosis process. Do the exercise while in a comfortable position. Obviously comfort facilitates relaxation. To maximize your relaxation experience lie down on a couch or the floor, or sit in a large chair that supports your head. Make sure your feet and legs are comfortable. Take off your glasses and shoes. Loosen or remove any restrictive articles of clothing or jewelry. Have a blanket available to cover you if necessary (you will want to stay warm). Put on some pleasant, relaxing music.

DIRECT SUGGESTION AND BODY AREA FOCUS

Relaxation can be achieved through direct suggestion. The body responds to requests that we give it. If you tell yourself enough times that you feel relaxed, you will start to actually relax. This is fairly simple to do. Basically, just suggest to yourself that your body is relaxed. The key words that work well for most people are "warm," "heavy," and "relaxed." Repeat those words over and over, "My body feels warm, heavy, and relaxed." It is useful to focus your suggestion initially on specific body parts, especially the large muscle masses of the arms and legs. Tell your arms that they are feeling warm, heavy and relaxed. Then tell your legs that they are feeling warm, heavy, and relaxed. Move on to other body parts, focusing on one area at a time, such as feet, calves, thighs, then the entire leg. Repeat the phrase several times for each area, stopping to notice the feelings in that area for five to ten seconds. Your feelings may include tingling, warmth, heaviness, muscular relaxation, and other pleasant sensations. Direct your suggestions of relaxation to parts of the body where it will be believable. If you tend to have cold hands and feet, you may want to attend to those areas later, after first relaxing the arms and legs.

DIRECT SUGGESTION AND WHOLE BODY RELAXATION

It also feels good to relax the entire body. After you have practiced focusing on specific areas of your body, you can begin to practice whole body relaxation. Start at your toes and work up to the top of your head, relaxing each area of your body step by step. First, lying down or sitting, get comfortable. Then take several deep, releasing breaths. Begin to bring your awareness to your toes, feet, and ankles. Take a deep breath and tell this area of your body that it feels warm, heavy, and relaxed. Imagine that the joints and muscles are letting go. Your joints are releasing and your muscles are melting. Speak to those areas and take a few moments to really feel them. Move up to your calves, knees, thighs, and hip joints, and tell them that they feel warm, heavy, and relaxed. Imagine that the joints are releasing and the muscles are melting. Speak to them and feel them releasing and melting. Repeat this at the region of your pelvis and lower abdomen. Then your lower back. Then your chest and upper back. Then your fingers, hands, and wrists. Then your forearm, elbows, and shoulders. Then your head, neck, and face, focusing on your mouth, eyes, eyebrows, forehead, ears, and scalp. Then relax your entire body. As you are moving through your body, tell each part that it feels warm, heavy, and relaxed. Imagine all your joints releasing and stretching out comfortably, and all your muscles melting. Feel your body fully. When you have gone through your whole body (five to ten minutes), you can repeat the process or just lie there, focusing on how deeply calm your entire body feels. This is a great practice for learning how to relax more deeply. It can also be very helpful with insomnia. Often by the time you get to your head you will be asleep if you do this practice at night in bed.

Deepening Techniques

In addition to relaxation there are a number of other important deepening strategies that we can use to take us further into a transformational state. Although relaxation is very helpful in its own right and a common ingredient in hypnotic process, it is often used as a transition into other deepening methods. The relaxation process is more physical, more body-oriented than other methods. Focusing on relaxation can keep you peripherally aware of your physical body, which can limit the deepening experience. In hypnosis we want to leave body awareness behind and drop into a deeper, more absorbed mind space. After relaxing, we want to go deeper where experience is less constrained by time and space. In this section we will look at additional mind-oriented methods for deepening. Try each one and see which one you enjoy the most.

DIRECT SUGGESTION

It always strikes me as somewhat incredible that the human mind responds to a suggestion as nebulous as "go deeper," yet it does. A simple direct suggestion for deepening our self-hypnosis is, "I am going deeper and deeper." As a result of that statement you will find yourself going into a quiet place that is more internal. You can employ any equivalent phrase, such as, "I am going deeper and deeper into peace/comfort/heaviness/quiet." Hypnotists used to say "deeper into sleep," but I personally do not like to associate hypnosis with sleep. Sleep and the hypnotic state are very different from each other. Some people like the phrase "higher and higher." That is fine. It is a good idea to be consistent, however, in your phrasing and imagery. Since a lot of the imagery has to do with floating down, and relaxation wording refers to being heavy and relaxed, the idea of going deeper has a certain logic to it. As long as there is some consistency to your pattern, you can choose whatever wording feels best to you. Trust your feelings. Explore and find what works for you.

COUNTING DOWN

Another common method for relaxation and deepening is counting down. You may have seen a television program in which a hypnotist was counting backward from one hundred to one. This is actually a useful method, not just a television act. In self-hypnosis you can count from fifty to one, twenty to one, or ten to one. It just depends on how much time you have. Count one number down with each exhale, breathing slowly and deeply. This gives a natural rhythm to your counting. As you count occasionally tell yourself mentally, "With every number down I am becoming more and more relaxed," or, "I am going deeper inside." With practice your mind and body will become accustomed to going into an inner state as you count down. You can begin training your mind for this response by counting down from one hundred to one or fifty to one. Every few weeks reduce the count by ten until you are counting down from twenty to one. You can also use ten to one as your count for quicker sessions when you need to. Your mind will become used to this deepening method and will be able to attain a deeper state of comfort easily as you count down. Counting down is a very effective way to combine the wording for relaxation and deepening at the same time.

Another useful method is to count down rapidly from one hundred to one. Imagine you are riding an express elevator down to the deepest level of a subterranean learning center. Tell yourself before you begin that with every number down you will become more and more profoundly relaxed and deep. Using words like "profoundly relaxed" opens up your mind to new possibilities, and allows you to experience sensations you have never felt before. You can also use a sound cue, like a metronome or a noisy clock, one with a substantial tick-tock quality. Place it near you when you do your self-hypnosis. Tell yourself that the sound of the metronome or clock will take you deeper and deeper inside. You can count down with every tock or just listen to it with the intention that the passing of each moment will take you deeper.

VISUAL IMAGERY

Imagery is a very useful tool for deepening. There are three ways we can use visual imagery for that purpose. These are images that facilitate deep relaxation or relaxation images, images that give the mind a sense of going inside or going deep or deepening, and images that set the context for transformational suggestion or what we could call workspace images. These three approaches can be used independently or in combination. If your objective in a session or with a particular issue is to cultivate greater skill with relaxation, then you can emphasize the relaxation imagery. For brief sessions you can use the workspace imagery. Generally, however, combining all three together is good practice. One approach is to begin with deepening images that transport you to your special transformational workspace. That workspace can possess qualities that enhance physical and mental relaxation. In this way the imagery prepares body, mind, and transformational process simultaneously. The bottom line is to make the images work for you. Note that many of the images provided here use dreamlike content. This is because one of the goals is to increase creativity and dreamlike thinking. If realistic images are more desirable, that is also fine. Use the approach that works best for you.

Relaxation Images

Imagery can be used for deepening relaxation. One effective approach is to think of some relaxing, pleasant experience you have had. This might be sitting in front of a crackling fire. It could be soaking in a hot tub. Perhaps it is lying in bed with fresh flannel sheets, or sitting in the forest by a stream in the sunlight. Using an actual experience is an effective way to access relaxation. Remembering the experience brings back the feelings of that moment, including the way your body felt, helping you to access a sense of deep physical and mental relaxation. If no relaxing memories come to mind then you can create a pleasant mental image. Any relaxing images will work. With your eyes closed, imagine yourself in a warm pool, sitting in a mountain meadow, floating on a cloud, melting into warm sand, anything you like. Just pick something that makes you feel happy, comfortable, safe, and relaxed. Relaxation images can easily be integrated with deepening images. You could, for example, walk or float down to a relaxing place, such as slowly walking down steps into a warm pool.

Deepening Images

Deepening images often possess a quality of movement, such as descending a stairway or walking down a forest path. You can also use images of things that are sinking or floating down, circling, or moving slowly and rhythmically, such as a pearl sinking down in warm water, a leaf circling down to the earth, or waves washing gently over the beach. The following deepening imagery patterns are themes that my clients enjoy.

Play with them to find the ones that work well for you or create your own unique forms. You can use any images you like, calming images with a quality of floating, descending, or going inside.

CANYON WALLS—You are walking down into a canyon. The air is fresh, filled with the scent of pine. The red walls feel smooth and warm. It is very quiet. Far below you the blue-green thread of the river flows gently. Hearing the sound of a bird you look up to see a hawk circling over the canyon. It descends slowly, going deeper and deeper into the canyon with you.

CLIFFS—You are high above the cliffs along the water's edge. With your feathered wings you float on the warm updrafts of wind rising off cliff walls. The ocean is below you, each wave washing onto the vast expanse of beach. You soar effortlessly for miles with the warm wind under your wings. After flying for some time, you find a beautiful valley, a very magical place. You slowly circle down and descend into the valley.

EXPRESS ELEVATOR—You are in an elevator at the top of a skyscraper. You insert a special key and watch the numbers of the floors as the elevator begins to go down. It is a very fast express elevator. You feel yourself going down, going deeper. The elevator moves amazingly fast. It passes the first floor and continues descending. You finally reach the very deepest subterranean level, where your private workspace is located. You get out and enter a brilliant crystalline cavern far beneath the earth.

LEAVES AND FEATHERS—You watch the leaf (feather, drop of rain, snowflake) floating down to the earth. It descends slowly, moving down deeper and deeper, just floating.

FOREST PATH—Walking down the beautiful forest path, you feel joyful. You can hear a stream flowing in the distance and birds singing in the trees above. Warm sunlight pours down gently upon you. You continue hiking deeper into the forest. You are on your way to visit your friend, a wise old sage. You know that this is a very significant journey for you. On this journey you will receive important information and profound healing. You feel the changes already beginning to happen. You continue to go deeper and deeper into the forest.

LIGHT SPHERE—You are inside a giant sphere of light. This sphere is floating down in a beautifully colored world of vast plateaus and deep canyons. The light sphere bounces gently from one level to the next as you sink deeper and deeper into this place of deep peace. Far below is a brilliant light. You are heading to the very heart of the light.

OCEAN OF BLISS—You are floating in an ocean of bliss. It is your favorite color, and the temperature is amazingly comfortable. It is a place where there is no time or space; it just is, perfect. There is a wonderful fragrance in the air of jasmine (or rose). You just float. You are floating in that ecstatic, peaceful place. It is a wonderful place. Time has no meaning here. Direction and space have no meaning here. You just float in the warm liquid light as the soft colors wash over you and through you.

PEARL—You watch a pearl floating down in the warm blue water. You can see the soft colors of the water. You dive down deeper to watch the pearl sink. The water is a perfect temperature. You slowly sink down deeper and deeper. A dolphin appears to swim with you. You hold on to its back, and it carries you deeper, following the pearl. It is peaceful here, so very, very peaceful.

STAIRS—You are walking down a set of beautiful stairs. They lead into a garden (or a warm pool, or liquid light). The stairs are very beautiful, warm red brick against a wall covered with green ivy. The old brass rail is worn perfectly smooth. You feel that you are going deeper and deeper into an amazing place of healing. You feel your power growing.

Workspace Images

The final deepening images are workspace images. These are images of a place you enter to do your transformational process. If you use this imagery consistently it will become identified with change. It can then be used for quick self-hypnosis sessions, by just imaging that space and giving yourself your suggestions there. The space can be real or fanciful. Fanciful imagery can be useful as it encourages a creative, dreamlike experience. Whatever space you choose it should be safe, peaceful, absent of extraneous people, and designed for imagery processing. It can be a secret mountain cavern, a tropical grotto, a tree house, a top-secret underground command center, the inside of a star, whatever captures your attention. It should have one or two comfortable places to sit or recline. It also needs something like a movie screen that is used for watching yourself doing your target behavior successfully. This viewing area can be a movie screen, crystal, a forest pond, an energy field; be creative. It can be fun creating this space. Once constructed, you can go there, see yourself looking very comfortable, and then use the movie screen to observe yourself being successful at your target behavior. This can become a useful component of successful self-hypnosis.

HYPNOTIC PHENOMENA

Hypnotic phenomena are a specific set of perceptual and behavioral experiences that can occur spontaneously during hypnosis, and that also can be intentionally evoked to deepen the state. These phenomena are natural to the human experience. They include age regression, amnesia, analgesia, automatic behavior, catalepsy, dissociation, hallucination, ideomotor behavior, posthypnotic suggestion, proprioceptive distortion, and time distortion.

Although it might not be immediately obvious, we do commonly experience many of these phenomena through the course of a week. For example, do you ever think you hear the phone ringing while you are in the shower (and it is not ringing)? That is auditory hallucination. Have you ever lost track of time during a good movie? That is time distortion. What about forgetting to buy the milk when you go to the store, the one thing you really needed? Amnesia. Have you ever had memories of your own childhood when you heard a child laugh or cry? That is age regression. All of these normally occurring perceptual shifts are used in hypnosis. In that context they are known as hypnotic phenomena. They are useful in hypnosis as they help elicit the appropriate mind and body states and can therefore significantly enhance deepening. They are one of the things that make hypnosis different from other methods used to transform beliefs. The fact that we have these experiences and can use them intentionally to evoke a special state of mind and body is interesting in its own right. So let us take a quick look at creating or eliciting hypnotic phenomena for the sake of deepening the hypnotic state.

GENERAL PRINCIPLES

There are two ways to deepen your hypnotic experience with hypnotic phenomena. The first way is to give yourself the suggestion that you will go deeper inside as the hypnotic phenomena occurs. For example, "As my eyelids become fused together (the hypnotic phenomena of catalepsy), I go deeper and deeper into my place of healing/vision/power." This is pairing together the idea of deepening with the experience of the hypnotic phenomena. The second way to deepen your experience is to test the phenomena. Using the eyelids example again, if you tried to open your locked eyelids and could not, you would go more deeply into hypnosis. Deepening occurs in that case because the test (trying to open your eyes and being unable to do so) provides a confirmation to your mind that you are now in an altered state.

HYPNOTIC PHENOMENA TECHNIQUES

Examples of specific hypnotic phenomena follow. Each one includes a technique for you to try. See which ones work best for you. Like everything else in life, people differ in terms of how they respond to these practices. All of them are fascinating and effective for deepening. When you use these hypnotic phenomena remember to finish your session by telling yourself that the phenomena are released. Just give your mind the opposite directions from those you used to create the hypnotic phenomena effect, such as, "My eyelids now open easily and feel wonderful." Probably nothing would happen if you did not undo the phenomena, but it is a good practice to undo them. That practice helps to make the phenomena more event related.

Age Regression

In age regression you reexperience something from your past. That past could be yesterday or forty years ago. The depth of the regression will determine the vividness of your memory experience. It is common to remember things you have not thought about for years. You may reexperience the original moment as if you were there. It can be quite amazing. (Probably the most amazing thing about it is that so much life data is stored away in us somewhere.) Regression can be useful for remembering positive things about our lives, for reworking stuck areas and limiting experiences, and for creating a healthier past image. I was recently working with a fifty-three year old client. She had an extremely vivid experience of being back in her childhood home in Holland, seeing people and places long forgotten. It was very positive and powerful for her. If you really need to work with strong negative memories and experiences from the past you will be better served by doing that with the assistance of a licensed psychotherapist who practices hypnosis. Do not do that work on your own as access to negative past experiences can be disturbing.

TECHNIQUE—One useful regression method is an equivalent feeling regression. In this method you go back into a past experience that elicits a specific feeling that would be useful right now. For example, whenever I need to feel persistence and increased energy I remember a time when I was running down the narrow mountain paths of Castle Crag Park. It was a hot summer day, and I felt absolutely incredible, a total peak experience. I go back to a specific memory of that run (that is a regression), and I instantly feel more power in my body, more vitality, passion, and a willingness to keep going. Invoking the memory invokes the feeling. It is a very useful strategy for quick boosts, such as before an athletic performance, an exam, or a cold call. Use a memory of something you are very good at, something fun. I often think of a specific moment of downhill skiing in Colorado, and that instantly puts me in a positive, powerful mind-body space. Find a memory that empowers you and use it when you need to get activated. Remember a past episode of courage, strength, or compassion, any memory of a success that evokes the appropriate feeling that you need right now. Really get into the memory for a moment. Once remembered, you will be in that state. As a general strategy, before you do anything important, access a powerful success memory and get into a success state.

Amnesia

Amnesia is the inability to recall something. In therapy, for example, when a person comes out of a deep hypnosis session they often will not remember anything that was said to them during the session. They were not asleep, as they come right back when you ask them to return to normal conscious awareness. (You can always tell when a client falls asleep, and you gently awaken them to continue since the sleeping mind is not very receptive.) When you inquire as to what happened during the session, they recall little or nothing because they were in a deep state. This is like someone daydreaming in class while the teacher is discussing the homework assignment. When the teacher asks that student to repeat the assignment, there is no response. The student was mentally inside somewhere. Although amnesia is used more commonly in conventional hypnosis than in self-hypnosis, it can be useful as a deepening tool.

TECHNIQUE—Tell yourself as you are beginning your deepening that you do not remember the number three, and that your inability to remember the number three will take you into a deeper space inside. Repeat this suggestion several times. Count down mentally from ten to one as your deepening method. If your mind responds easily to amnesia, you will not remember the number three as you count to one. If you prefer, tell yourself that you cannot remember the day or month. This helps take your mind out of linear time. This method can also be useful to help break a habit pattern. For example, if someone smoked when on a coffee break, amnesia could be used to suggest that when on their break they will not remember that they smoke cigarettes. It sounds funny, but it can work.

Anesthesia and Analgesia

Anesthesia is the removal of sensation. Novocaine at the dentist's office is an anesthetic. Analgesia is the removal of pain. An aspirin is an analgesic. With an analgesic you can feel other sensations, such as warmth and vibration, but you do not feel pain. Hypnosis can create both types of sensory modifications. These experiences also occur naturally, for example when your arm falls asleep after you have been lying on it, leaving you with minimal sensation, or when a runner goes far enough to activate a runner's high. At such times the body does not feel much discomfort or pain. These are examples of a normal mind-body capacity. Although this method is more useful as a hypnotic treatment for pain, it can also be used for deepening. We will come back to it when we talk about pain control in the applications section in chapter 12.

TECHNIQUE—Place your hands on your thighs if sitting or next to your body if lying down. Tell yourself as you are deepening that your hands are becoming so heavy that they are dissolving. You can no longer feel them. Keep repeating to yourself that they are becoming more relaxed and heavy, that they are just dissolving. You are unable to feel them. They have no sensation. They are heavy and numb. They are gone. Repeat these suggestions with each exhale. Allow your hands to become profoundly heavy and to dissolve. They become large stones, heavy, without sensation, sinking down into the earth. Tell your hands they will feel better than ever when you return.

Automatic Behavior

Automatic behavior includes automatic writing, sleep walking, spontaneous movements, channeling, speaking in tongues, and related activities. In automatic behavior the inner mind moves the body, speaks, writes, and performs other actions. It might appear that the person is consciously controlling the behavior, but it is not conscious. The behavior is an automatic, unconscious process. It is not intentional or controlled. It just happens. One form of automatic behavior that works very well for self-hypnosis is automatic movement. That will be discussed more in a moment when we examine ideomotor movement. Another automatic behavior that I find useful (not for deepening, but rather for insight) is to have my inner mind ask me questions out loud. I can then answer the questions. My answers often provide valuable insight as they are answers to questions I would not normally have thought to ask. This often provides an entirely different perspective and thus new insights. It can be a very helpful method.

TECHNIQUE—To gain automatic answers, just sit with your eyes closed and go into a quiet space. Let your inner voice ask a question (out loud) as if it were the voice of an inner sage, a being of great compassion and wisdom. Then answer the question out loud or write down the answer.

Catalepsy

Catalepsy is a form of paralysis. It is a very powerful form of deepening. The inability to open your eyelids when they are hypnotically fused together is an example of catalepsy (refer to the inductions in chapter 7). When our eyes are stuck shut and we try to open them unsuccessfully, we get confirming evidence that we are in an altered state, so our state goes deeper. Catalepsy can be applied to any body part or to the entire body.

TECHNIQUE—If you are doing hypnosis in a seated position, it can be interesting to make your lower body immobile. To do this, tell yourself that you feet are becoming fixed to the floor. Feel them become heavy and immovable. As they do this, tell yourself that you are going deeper into hypnosis. Try to lift your feet to test this deepening. If you are lying down, tell yourself that your entire body is getting more and more rigid, immovable. Feel yourself deepening as your body becomes more rigid.

Dissociation

Dissociation is experiencing your mind, body, or feelings as separate from your self. This can be a useful phenomenon for working with pain, getting perspective on issues, or analyzing problems more dispassionately.

In this method you would take some body part, feeling, or thought and separate it from you, perhaps placing it a few feet away from you. You can then look at it and tell yourself you are going deeper as you experience that part of yourself as separate. You can also see your entire body in another location.

TECHNIQUE—First imagine that your physical body is floating on warm water. Then let your mental body float down out of your physical body. Look up at your physical body and watch it get smaller and smaller as you float further down. Let your emotional body drop down out of your mental body. Watch your mental body get smaller and smaller as your emotional body sinks further down into warmth and peace. You can still see your physical body far above your mental body as a tiny point of light.

If you prefer, sit in a chair or lie down, close your eyes, and see an image of yourself sitting next to you. The one sitting next to you is doing the hypnosis session on you. You become the hypnotist and the client at the same time. Alternatively, see yourself on television. Watch your televised self perfectly performing your desired outcome behaviors, driving the car you want, looking healthy and successful, winning a gold medal, whatever your heart desires.

Hallucination—Positive and Negative

A hallucination is a sensory misperception. Hallucinations can be in any sensory channel. You can hallucinate olfactory, gustatory, visual, auditory, and kinesthetic experiences. A positive hallucination involves experiencing a sensation, such as a smelling, hearing, or seeing something, when in actuality there is nothing there. A negative hallucination is the inability to experience something that actually is there. An example of a positive hallucination would be smelling an orange being peeled when no orange is present. The more real the smell appears to be the stronger the hallucination. I worked with someone once who experienced an extremely vivid smell of jasmine while in hypnosis. She thought I had sprayed something in the air. It was late winter and there was no jasmine or jasmine scent present. Interestingly, we were doing regression for her to recall her grandmother whom she loved very much. Jasmine was her beloved grandmother's favorite flower. A negative hallucination, by contrast, is the removal of a sensory object. As an example, I once induced a negative visual hallucination for a client in which he could not see for a few minutes. That was very compelling evidence that hypnosis works, which is why he wanted to do such an unusual exercise.

TECHNIQUE—Tell yourself as you are deepening that you are having a vivid experience of some specific taste, smell, sound, touch, or image. Pick a sense channel that is strong for you, and then pick an experience with that sense that you enjoy. You might hear a loving voice, reassuring and comforting you. Smell a pleasant flower or feel a warm breeze on your face. Tell your mind that are going deeper as you imagine your experience.

Ideomotor Behavior

We have already played with ideomotor processes back in chapter 7 when we worked with hands moving together as an induction method. Ideomotor processes are very powerful. Ideomotor behavior essentially means that an idea, or suggestion, becomes movement. Ideomotor methods invoke the inner mind to move the body, such as elevating an arm. The movement carries you deeper as it presents very tangible evidence that something non-normal is occurring.

TECHNIQUE—A nice ideomotor exercise, Hands Moving Together, can be found in chapter 7.

Posthypnotic Suggestion

Posthypnotic suggestions are secondary suggestions that can help increase the effect of our primary hypnotic suggestions. They work by providing cues or triggers to reactivate our primary suggestions when we need them. We give ourselves both types of suggestions during our hypnosis session. For example, you can use a hypnotically suggested trigger stimuli, such as seeing the clock on the wall in the classroom, to remind you to stay calm during an exam. In this case the posthypnotic suggestion given in hypnosis would be, "When I see the clock on the wall during the exam, I will feel deeply relaxed and confident." The suggestion is that during the exam, a clock will trigger (posthypnotic suggestion) the relaxation and confidence we are suggesting (primary hypnotic suggestion). We will examine the process of posthypnotic suggestions in more detail in the upcoming chapter on concluding a session.

Proprioceptive Distortion

Proprioceptive distortion is the sense that your body is different in some way from its actual size or position. These distortions can include changes in the perceived location of your body; perceived movements, like swaying or spinning motions; and an experience of alteration in the size of your body or your body parts, such as having very large hands or a large head.

TECHNIQUE—Tell yourself as you deepen that your body is floating down and you feel yourself falling backward slowly into a very deep ocean of light. You are falling backwards and slowly spiraling down a long tunnel of light. You will be amazed to feel yourself floating down backward in a vast arc through space, like a slow-motion dive that never ends.

Time Distortion

Time distortion uses the subjective experience of the passage of time to alter consciousness. If we can lose track of time we have one less reference to the linear world of our conscious mind. In the dream world, time has little meaning. Experiences of things long past or future years away are as viable as the present moment. In hypnosis we use this natural capacity of the mind to play with both the direction and the pace of time to help us go more deeply into a creative learning space. This can make a relatively brief session feel much longer, infinitely long even.

TECHNIQUE—Tell yourself that you no longer know what day it is, what time it is, what month it is. Tell yourself that you feel like you have been in deep hypnosis for a long, long time. You may experience the eternal. It is always right here if you can find it and open to it. Just repeat to yourself that you are in an expansive, timeless place.

Creating Safety

It is important to create a sense of safety if you plan on working very deeply. A sense of safety will enable you to let go and explore openly. You can use whatever method you prefer for creating this sense, such as surrounding yourself with light, stating that you will have a completely positive healing experience, or working with an ally. The latter can be a powerful method. If you work with an ally, such as an angel, then have that angel be with you, perhaps holding a golden strand attached to your ankle, during your session. I use that method for some of my deepest work. The bottom line is to create a sense of safety and comfort in doing your work so that you can make progress comfortably. Always emphasize that you are going to have deeply positive experiences. Finally, remember to be prudent. Despite how hypnosis is often portrayed in the media, trancework needs to be approached wisely and respectfully. It is a powerful tool that can confer great benefit to those who use it well. It is also no replacement for professional help when dealing with with complex, painful issues.

Practice Notes

Jot down your experiences and insights from trying various deepening techniques. What worked best for you?

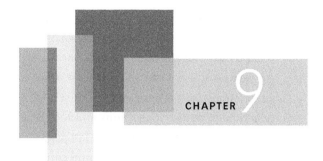

CHAPTER 9

using hypnotic suggestions— *transforming*

Visioning

Focusing

Deepening

Transforming

Concluding

In the previous chapters we learned how to prepare the energy field of mind and body. Working with vision, induction, relaxation, and deepening, we accessed a creative inner hypnotic space and increased our receptivity to powerful new ideas. The next thing we will learn is how to create effective suggestions to put into that powerful energy field.

Hypnotic Suggestions

In the Focusing chapter we learned about entering the house of transformation. In the Deepening chapter we learned about going further into the house and sitting in a comfortable chair in front of the fireplace. In this chapter on Transforming we will learn how to use hypnotic suggestions to weave a story of our successful life as we sit in that chair. High-quality suggestions are a critical element of self-hypnosis. In this chapter we will examine hypnotic suggestions and look at how to construct a comprehensive approach using positive language, visual imagery, direct suggestions, posthypnotic suggestions, and concluding suggestions.

Gain with No Pain

One of the unique things about hypnotic suggestions, something that can take time to truly appreciate, is that they produce change effortlessly. Once the hypnotic suggestion is presented to the receptive learning space, your mind-body energy field takes over. It begins working to find the necessary inspiration, energy, commitment, and solutions to your issues. That inner process generates insights, and new patterns begin to emerge. You find yourself changing, seeing things differently and behaving more powerfully; your goal starts to move toward you.

Everyone has probably had the experience of studying or practicing some skill, such as playing the piano or doing math, and then putting it aside for a while. When you came back to it months later you found that you had improved somehow. Something integrated the knowledge inside you during that time. Even though it was not a conscious process, during that interim you learned new things and grew from that. It all happened beneath the surface without conscious effort. That is how hypnotic suggestion works.

I remember a humorous personal experience that showed me the power of hypnotic suggestion. I was teaching a class on hypnotherapy. Two of my students were doing a hypnotic double induction on me. My request was to receive suggestions that would help me to get up earlier and to exercise more. They began their inductions, and in no time I was in a deep hypnotic state. When they brought me back I had no recollection of anything they had told me. They looked at each other mischievously and laughed. I did too. Well the next morning before the alarm went off, I jumped out of bed at 5:00 a.m. and decided it would be a good morning for a bike ride. I got on my bike and rode down to the beach. I proceeded to jump in and go for a swim (which is pretty crazy at 5:30 in the morning as the ocean is very cold around here). Well that intensity lasted for a little less than a week before it began to even out. In a later conversation with one of the students, I was informed that they had given me suggestions to awaken early in the morning with a strong desire to bicycle and swim. That event made me an even stronger believer in the power of hypnosis to manifest positive changes and new insights without our conscious knowledge of the process or our conscious effort to change. In hypnosis the process does not have to be conscious. The change just happens. It comes about as a consequence of appropriate suggestions given to a deep inner energy field that is highly receptive to new learning and transformation.

Affirmations Compared to Hypnotic Suggestions

This notion of an unconscious or inner process suggests an important distinction between hypnosis and affirmation. Certainly affirmation practices are very powerful. I use them often myself. However, affirmations work more at the conscious level. We repeat the positive phrase in our conscious mind. The problem with that is that the conscious mind is not necessarily as open to new information. That mind is at the level that maintains our personal limiting beliefs about ourself via our inner critic, doubter, worrier, complainer, and similar voices. It logically defends and maintains those old patterned beliefs. That mind is the internal bureaucrat. It serves to maintain the status quo, even if that status quo is totally dysfunctional.

The deep mind that hypnosis accesses, however, is a more flexible and creative place. It is a dissecting, exploring, synthesizing, creating, learning mind. It functions like a child's mind, always building things up and breaking them down again in order to understand the universe. This mind can accept new ideas and work with them. It is like our dream mind in which all things are possible, where strange new things are believable and even embraced. When we place our suggestions or ideas in at that deep hypnotic level of mind and body, they meet with minimal resistance. They tap into a creative energy field that is helpful in generating new ways to reach our desired goals. That is the reason for using induction and deepening rather than just giving ourselves a conscious suggestion or affirmation. Conscious mind suggestions are useful, but generally they have more inertia to deal with, more bureaucracy, and consequently they are slower, less creative, and less productive than hypnotic suggestion.

Principles of Powerful Verbal Suggestions

We will examine three types of hypnotic suggestions—verbal, visual, and metaphoric. We can start by looking at how to build powerful verbal suggestions. A verbal suggestion is a word or a phrase. It is like an affirmation except that it is given to the deep mind in hypnosis. To create the best verbal suggestions, develop them with the following ideas in mind.

ADDRESS THE ISSUE

Make sure, to the extent you can know, that your suggestions match the issue and goal you are addressing. You should have a sense of the issue or problem's primary layer (as we discussed in chapter 6). It is important to base your goals on your deeper values as well. Refer to the visioning activities you did in chapter 6 on prioritizing your values. If your goals do not match your values, those goals can encounter inner resistance. Think of ideal outcomes.

Make your suggestions very specific. If you are a golfer, for example, give yourself specific suggestions regarding holding the club, using body flow, having a confident mental focus, and so on. If, however, you do not know exactly what you need or want, a more exploratory or open frame serves well. If you were trying to determine a career path, for example, and had no clear sense of what career you wanted to get into, then you could use more general suggestions. Rather than saying, "I will become a pharmacist," a person would use suggestions such as, "I am finding the career information I need, meeting people who provide me excellent career advice, getting greater career clarity, and making wise decisions. My deep mind will help me to know what my perfect career is. I know it now. I love the work I am going to be doing. It is perfect for me."

Always remember to be clear about your goals and go for the greatest good. You can ask for anything, but always keep in mind what really makes you happy. At the deepest level many of the things we think we want may be neurotic needs or symbolic of something else, something more subtle. The big car may be a need for respect. Wanting a partner may be a need to feel safe in the world. What we are really seeking is the symbolic benefit we derive from the car, person, wardrobe, house. It can be very helpful to look at our underlying need to determine what disguised benefits we are actually seeking. Often they are emotional needs of safety, self-respect, love, or happiness.

> It can be very helpful to look at our underlying need to determine what disguised benefits we are actually seeking. Often they are emotional needs of safety, self-respect, love, or happiness.

Once we recognize the underlying need, we can work directly on that issue, or work simultaneously on getting the car and building the sense of worthiness and respect at the same time. No matter what you ask for, it can be useful to include suggestions for those deeper foundation needs too: of love, health, peace, happiness, courage, power, wisdom, generosity, or abundance. Filling both sets of needs will help to provide more ultimately satisfying, healing, and empowering solutions, and a much richer life.

It is also useful to ask yourself whether you are really willing to remove the obstacles from your life to make something positive happen. If not, there may be little value in working on that goal now. If you are not quite ready for real change in your life, then hypnosis can be used as a preparatory process. If someone comes to me for hypnosis, to quit smoking for example, and I know they are not ready yet, then we work on getting ready to quit. We prepare them for quitting at some future point, rather than trying now and not succeeding. It is good to be honest about where you are at in your process and work on the appropriate level. Time heals.

USE POSITIVE WORDING

Generally we want to phrase our hypnotic suggestions positively. Which of the following sounds better to you? "I am really smart," or, "I'm not as dumb as I thought." Similar meaning, very different feeling. The same rule applies when we talk to ourselves or give ourselves suggestions. Be positive. Make a list of the things you want to change, improve, increase, or decrease. Remove any limiting terms and create a positive statement. Focus on the positive components. For examples, instead of saying, "I no longer eat so much junk food," say, "I now eat energizing, life-giving foods." Instead of saying, "My cancer is growing more slowly," say, "My healing energy gets stronger every day. Healthy cells grow and unhealthy energy leaves my body." Instead of saying, "People no longer reject me," say, "People love to be with me." Instead of, "I am not missing the ball," say, "My average is increasing steadily and will continue to rise during the season." Use an active, powerful, positive voice.

VARY THE PERSPECTIVE

Variety is the spice of life. Variety keeps the mind engaged. Similarly, it can be helpful to have several variations for your suggestions. You want to present the transformational suggestion to your mind from a number of perspectives. Generally, the more sides of an object we see, the more we understand what it is. Variety gives the inner mind more information to work with. Additionally, developing various suggestions means that you have thought about your goal in detail, which can only help. If you want to lose weight, for example, you can suggest that you eat healthy food, you eat light and energizing amounts of food, you exercise every day, your body gets lighter and stronger, you are happy, you love yourself, and others love you. Those suggestions would provide a comprehensive and varied palette of appropriately interrelated suggestions.

Creating variation in your suggestions may require you to understand your issue more completely. Information exists on virtually every subject today. Do not be shy. Resources exist to help you. You can even do your research at home on the Internet. Go to a bookstore in another town. Talk to a counselor. Call an information hotline. There is so much information available to offer insight. Knowledge can be very liberating. Often just knowing some facts about our concern can relieve fear and doubt. Get as much information as you can and incorporate the most relevant ideas into your hypnotic suggestions.

REPEAT SUGGESTIONS THROUGHOUT THE SESSION

During your session you will want to give yourself your hypnotic suggestion(s) repeatedly. Soon we will be putting all the parts together—relaxation, deepening, and transformational suggestion. During hypnosis you will just keep cycling through those three elements over and over again. The first two, relaxation and deepening, keep the deep mind open. The suggestion is then put into that creative energy field to generate empowered new beliefs, inspiration, and action. You will want to maintain all three aspects—relaxation, deepening, and suggestion—while in a session. Relaxation and deepening get you comfortably seated in front of the fireplace. Hypnotic suggestions weave the story. These two activities are the yin and yang of hypnosis. They need each other to be complete.

PRESENT AND FUTURE PERSPECTIVES

Generally we do self-hypnosis to move toward a desired goal. We can do it to explore the past, but even exploration of the past ideally serves to clear the path to an improved future. Exploring the past for its own sake is not the best use of self-hypnosis. Self-hypnosis is about solutions, moving forward. To this end it is important to phrase suggestions so they focus on the present and the future. For example, if you are dealing with personal money management and planning, you might rephrase the suggestion, "I am moving out of this debt," to "Money is flowing into my life now, and my savings and investments are significant and growing (present and future)."

We want to put ourselves into a successful picture, as if the future were here now. This helps to pull us forward toward our dream, our desired goal. Someone quitting drugs would want to see himself or herself looking successful now: clean, sober, healthy, and happy. It is important to phrase suggestions as if they were already true now. If we only used future phrases that would keep our outcomes in the future. Some suggestions should be phrased to reflect current success, "I am so happy now, my savings are bigger than ever." In addition, some suggestions should imply even greater future success, "My happiness will continue to grow as my love expands every day." By including some future-oriented phrases we create more expectancy for enduring and increasing success.

LIMIT THE NUMBER OF SUGGESTIONS

When we start doing transformational work, we sometimes get inspired and try to fix everything at once. That is like trying to balance too many plates at once. Ultimately each issue gets less attention with that approach. On the other hand, too little attention is like too little medicine. You need to take enough to get your desired results. Half the recommended dose does not produce half the effect, it often produces no effect. You need the right amount. So in each session concentrate on one topic or issue. You can do lots of quick sessions throughout the day, so the number of issues is potentially limitless. At any one sitting, however, focus on one major goal assignment.

PERSONALIZE THEM

If your suggestions come from an affirmation book that is acceptable. It is much better, however, to create your own. When you create suggestions with your own words and ideas, they will hold more power for you. Use your name in your suggestions. Use ideas that motivate you. If you value being a good parent, for example, and your issue is reducing procrastination, you can suggest, "I am becoming more focused and productive, and this is creating extra time and energy for me to be with my family." If you are a religious person, you could include ideas from your beliefs. This practice is called binding, associating the desired outcome with something important or motivating. I use it all the time when I work with clients. It can be very helpful. Another motivating strategy is to consider how a problematic issue actually obstructs your deepest goals and happiness. If we can see its toxicity in our lives that can be very, very motivating.

INCLUDE POSTHYPNOTIC SUGGESTION

Another important suggestion that can be given during a session is a posthypnotic suggestion (one of the hypnotic phenomena discussed in chapter 8). A posthypnotic suggestion increases the power of a session by retriggering key behaviors and feelings during the week. Give yourself a suggestion while in hypnosis that during the week, whenever you experience the trigger (your choice, something relevant but not too common), you will have a specific thought, feeling, or behavior that will help you with your transformational success. For example, if you wanted to quit smoking, you would tell yourself during the session, "Every time I hear the phone ring, I will feel totally enthusiastic about quitting smoking." This would be a good reinforcement trigger for someone who smoked while on the phone.

Pick a trigger that closely precedes the occurrence of your issue, like the phone ringing before picking up a cigarette for people who smoke while on the phone. In this way the hypnotically suggested trigger stimulates an appropriate response before the problematic behavior occurs. Also, try to select trigger that is related to the issue. For example, if one of your spouse's behaviors increases your anger and results in arguments, you can use one of his or her facial expressions (your preargument trigger) to elicit personal relaxation and perspective. If you are a performer you can use a specific body posture, such as standing tall and expanding your chest, as a pre-performance trigger for accessing the performance confidence that you worked on in your hypnosis. You can also use a more pervasive trigger, such as hearing the hour chime on your watch or seeing a stop sign, as a reminder to practice a more generalized behavior, such as learning to relax or feeling more prosperous.

Principles of Powerful Visual Suggestions

The second major type of hypnotic suggestion is visualizing desired outcomes. Visualizing is a process of seeing with the mind's eye. We experience this frequently throughout the day. We daydream. We see images of friends in our mind, images from last night's television program, images of our childhood triggered when we hear a youngster's laughter. It is a common everyday occurrence. It is also an effective tool for hypnotic transformation.

Just as we can use words to convey suggestions to the deep mind, we can also use images to convey suggestions. These are visual suggestions. When we use images of beaches and forest ponds to help us relax, that is called visual imagery. Visual imagery, as we have read earlier, is very effective for relaxation and deepening. However, when we use images that portray our desired outcome, that is what is referred to as a visual suggestion. For example, seeing an image in your mind of yourself driving the new car you want, you are making a visual suggestion to yourself. Using visual suggestions in this way is extremely useful because we can visualize anything we want, fanciful or real. There are no limits to what we can conceive mentally. That flexibility makes imagery a powerful tool for delivering hypnotic suggestions to ourselves.

The method of visualizing suggestion as described in this section will help you create an experience of your goal, the way it would look, sound, feel, smell, and taste. Because sensory images are more representative of reality than the words that describe them, they create a rich encounter with the goal. Recall the axiom, "One picture is worth a thousand words." With a visual suggestion you can get a valuable representation of what you want. Using visual suggestions in addition to verbal suggestions provides a very powerful combination for our transformational work.

WHY USE VISUAL IMAGES?

Humans rely heavily on visual information to know their environment. We are bipedal, binocular mammals. Vision has played a dramatic role in our evolutionary development. There are over fifteen million rods and cones in our retina that allow us to see colors, shapes, and movement. About 30 percent of the cortex of the human brain that's involved in sensory experience is related to vision. This is significantly more than any other sense modality, including touch. The visual sense has helped us become what we are as a species, and it continues to play a fundamental role in our existence. In contemporary society we surround ourselves with visual representations. We live in an immersive visual landscape of photographs, maps, diagrams, film, television, movies, written words, magazines, and books. From the time we are young children, we are taught extensively via the visual channel. Visual experience pervades the way we think and the way we know the world. It is a primary sensory reality.

One important benefit of visual imagery is that it is barrier free. You can see yourself doing impossible things, like flying to the sun on a winged horse. Shamanic work uses imagery to access novel insight. Because imagery transcends time boundaries, we can imagine the future as tangible. We can see ourselves running a marathon in a personal best record time, depositing large checks in the bank, closing the biggest deal ever, having a loving relationship, healing a serious illness. Seeing is believing. Imagery begins to create a pattern in our mind, a picture of possibilities. This image map lays a foundation for hope and positive expectancy. If we use imagery to increase our belief that something is possible, that belief begins to generate a positive self-fulfilling prophecy. Psychology research shows that human learning is strengthened by doing. Through imagery we can have an experience of doing anything—virtually. We can learn new things by enacting them in our mind. Through this inner doing we can experience success with new behaviors and other important goals. As a result of this virtual process, when we perform the actual behavior we will have already positively rehearsed and experienced it.

Imagery is also memorable. One picture is worth a thousand words. An image conveys a vast amount of information. It is compact. A religious icon is a single painting, yet it opens up a vast space of feelings and beliefs. It is a visual doorway to a much larger experience. It is easier to access one icon that represents one thousand things than it is to remember the thousand things themselves. For example, think of a wonderful vacation or some peak experience you had within the past few years. Close your eyes and go there. Get an image of that experience then notice your body-mind feelings. Remembering that image rekindles those feelings. Attaining that same state through a verbal description of the event would take more time and effort. The appropriate image can help us access powerful states on demand, like a light switch. Once you locate that switch, you can use it to turn powerful states on and off at will.

> Because imagery transcends time boundaries, we can imagine the future as tangible.

HOW TO CREATE A RICH VISUAL SUGGESTION

Visual suggestions take the desired outcome and turn it into an image. Instead of stating or describing our outcome in words, we use sensory images to build it. Creating effective visual suggestions relies on some basic principles—giving the image feeling, being specific, making the images present- and future-oriented, and being positive. The visual suggestions should be as sensory rich as possible, and they should include all the appropriate sensory elements (sound, touch, taste, and smell, as well as sight). As an example, imagine you had a goal of winning a marathon. You would create a comprehensive sensory display of that goal to incorporate into your session. That could include seeing yourself crossing the finish line ahead of all of the other runners, hearing the announcer calling out your name as the winner, feeling the exhilaration as you crossed the line, arms extended up into the air, and smelling the air as you slowed down and breathed in deeply. We want to make our outcome images vivid, as rich as life. The imagery should reflect the ultimate success you want to experience.

If your visual image is somewhat vague, that is fine. If for whatever reason it is not a clear picture or a strong feeling, start with whatever version comes to mind. If you only get a piece of a picture then work with that piece. You can take that bit of imagery and amplify it. Make it bigger, brighter, or louder. If you get no picture, then pretend. Ask yourself, "If it had an image, what would it look like?" This begins to build the image at some level in your mind, whether you can actually include it or not. Your desired outcome is still there affecting you. You can use this pretend strategy to create very elaborate representations, even if you have no success with visual imaging at this point. For example, you can augment imagery with words. Verbally describe the image to yourself and elaborate upon it. You can also draw images that reflect your goal or clip pictures from magazines. Work with concrete physical images to help you develop your own internal images. In time with practice, your skill in working with visual images will grow. It is a learnable skill.

I once had a student who could not create visual images at all, which was rare. I asked him to imagine an angel, while his eyes were closed. I asked, "What do you see." "Nothing." I then asked him, "If you could see it what would it look like?" He went on for several minutes describing in great detail what he "saw." The idea of the image was there somewhere. Imagery is not image dependent in my world of hypnosis. This is not religion. It is art. There is no right or wrong way. Just make it work for you.

GIVE THE IMAGE FEELING

Pairing strong feeling with your visual images makes them much more powerful. When two people see a picture of chocolate cake, one person may feel delight (the chocolate lover) while the other may feel disgust (the person allergic to chocolate). Same image, different feelings. It is the feeling that makes the imagery powerful. Images elicit feelings, and those feelings move people to act. If an image does not have a feeling associated with it, then we can predict it will not be very powerful, compelling, or motivating. If you see yourself winning the Olympic marathon but feel no joy or excitement, then it is not a very powerful or encouraging image. As you work with visual suggestions, you will learn that just visualizing something that you want does not necessarily produce feelings of desire for that outcome. This is probably even more true when the visual suggestion is one that you find hard to believe in or that you have minimal personal experience with. Especially in those cases it is incumbent on the visualizer to bring the appropriate feeling into the picture. It will become evident over time that images paired with strong corresponding emotion have more energy and consequently more impact. Bring your images to life with strong feelings. Allow yourself to believe in yourself and your goal. Hold the conviction in your heart that your vision is going to come true. Leave no room for doubt. Act as though it were guaranteed. Believe in your dream completely and get inspired.

> By visualizing exactly what you want during self-hypnosis, you are creating a powerful dream. It will begin to be reflected in your thoughts, words, and actions, moving you toward your goals.

BE SPECIFIC

Constructing a clear image of what you want will help you manifest your outcome. If you want to live in a bigger house then create that specific house in your mind: see it, believe it. By visualizing exactly what you want during self-hypnosis, you are creating a powerful dream. It will begin to be reflected in your thoughts, words, and actions, moving you toward your goals. The universe can hear your request and will support you and your dream, shaping that vibration into a new manifest reality. To be vague with your visual imagery suggestion can be a quiet statement of unworthiness or self-doubt. Allowing yourself to behold your dream is a statement to yourself: "I deserve to be happy, and I am ready to be happy." Clarity and specificity are power. Be honest about what you want. See what you want exactly the way you want it. Embrace it.

USE PRESENT AND FUTURE PERSPECTIVES

See your visions as current realities. Also see yourself six months or several years out in the future even more embodied with your goal. A simple self-hypnosis practice that you can use at times is to visualize your desired future life. Envision doing, having, or being the life you dream of. That future image begins to draw you to it. It becomes a self-fulfilling prophecy. Seeing is believing. A clear vision of our future helps us begin to believe that our goals are possible. This also makes us think more clearly about where we want to go. It is a very useful process. Do occasional sessions in which you clearly visualize what you want your life to look like in the future. See your amazing life as real, tangible, and manifested.

PRACTICE PERFECTLY

When you use visual images in self-hypnosis, you will want to see yourself doing the outcome perfectly. Give yourself room to be successful in your own mind. That alone is a good exercise for many people. Let the image be a success image. See the ideal outcome. It is not practice that makes perfect, it is correct practice that makes perfect.

PERSONALIZE IT

Make sure you are in your images, winning the race, getting the raise, being in love. Personalize your visual images, be associated with the image, be in it clearly. Let it be real for you, as if you were already there in that positive experience.

USE POSITIVE IMAGES

Always use positive, success-oriented images. See yourself as a complete success at whatever the desired outcome is. Let it be an inspiring image. We do negative self-hypnosis throughout the day when we entertain critical thoughts, fear, and images of failure or imperfection. The value of such thoughts is that they can give us a good window into our limiting beliefs, and as such can guide our choice of transformative imagery. It is simply a matter of taking one of those negative self-images and creating the reverse image. To start notice the negative pattern for a while, a few days or weeks. Maybe take some notes. Think of what that image looks like, how it behaves, what the feeling is inside the image, what drives it. When you have enough information then think of what the opposite of all of that would be. What would be the opposite therapeutic, transformational antidote to that negative self-imagery? Spend some time getting clear on that antidote imagery as well. Create that counterimage and use it in your self-hypnosis session. Use self-hypnosis to get into the quiet, peaceful state and then bring in the positive new self image. See it, be it, integrate it. Or you can just forget about the negative content and start from scratch. Build an ideal outcome image from the ground up, making it exactly what you want it to be. Do not be humble or hold back. This is the movie of your body-mind. This is your dream. Let it be as positive and powerful as it can realistically be. Have fun with the process. Fun is liberating.

Principles of Powerful Metaphoric Suggestions

The third main type of hypnotic suggestion is metaphoric. A metaphor is a word or idea or image used as a resemblance of something to help describe it, understand it, or work with it. The prefix *meta* means, among other things, change, as in metamorphosis. You change something ineffable, like the concept of God or Goddess for example, into something tangible, like Krishna, Jesus, or Kuan Yin. So a metaphor is a way to represent something (often abstract) as something else (often more concrete) in order to understand it better. Joseph Campbell, the great scholar of world mythology, spoke at length about how the world's ancient myths are metaphors for something more transpersonal and universal. The mythic masks, totems, rituals, and deities are metaphoric expressions of something more intangible and difficult to comprehend. So our human mind creates these metaphoric representations, such as deity images, to help us understand and relate to the mystery of life more fully.

Similarly, in hypnosis we can use stories and images metaphorically to convey more complex or abstract suggestions to our inner mind. For example, let us say that you needed a sense of security and protection in your life. You could use a description or an image of a bear as a metaphor for a protective quality to guard over you. That bear could then be incorporated into hypnotic imagery, being at your side, warding off negative forces. The key is to come up with images of things that represent the essence of the solution quality you are looking for. If you need courage bring in a lion, if you need fun bring in an otter, if you need healing bring in the sun. Let these forces be with you, talk to you, and guide you, or become them and feel their wisdom within you. This is a powerful tool available to us all.

Metaphoric suggestions are also helpful as tools for providing new perspectives and insight. As an example, say you wanted to do very well in a sporting event, like speed skating. You could become an arrow in your self-hypnosis session. You would then feel what it would be like to be streamlined, cutting through the air, moving with total concentration toward the bull's eye. That experience would provide you with new information about speed and focus. Such information is different from just imagining yourself skating fast and winning the race. The metaphoric image does not picture skating. It is an experience of an aspect of skating. It provides a new perspective that provides new information. You can learn new things this way and gain knowledge others may not possess. The ancient shamans learned from animals by becoming the animal. Through this process they came to understand an animal and its powers deeply. Metaphor used in this way can offer us very important insight into life.

Concluding Thought

By using verbal, visual, and metaphoric suggestions in your self-hypnosis practice, you have a variety of ways of inputting transformational content into your receptive body-mind energy field. These suggestions are highly flexible and powerful tools. With time your ability to create strong and effective hypnotic suggestions will grow, and you will be amazed at what they can offer.

Create Sample Hypnotic Suggestions

With the information in this chapter fresh in your mind, take a moment to create some working hypnotic suggestions.

VERBAL SUGGESTION

A verbal suggestion should say what you really want to experience. Do not be shy or modest. Do not hold back. Make it bold.

Create a verbal hypnotic suggestion addressing your goal in a personal and positive way, with a present and a future perspective. What kinds of things would your perfect coaches say if they were talking about you and the ideal outcome of your goal? Consider those expressions and write them down as "I" statements.

_____

_____

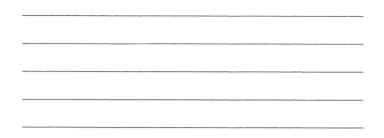

VISUAL SUGGESTION

The visual suggestion should be a clear image or movie of what you want your life to look like, exactly. Be powerful in your images. Make them reflect the dream you want. Think boldly.

Describe your ideal outcome as if you were there in it—sights, sounds, smells, whatever would make it very real. What would you be experiencing? How would you be feeling in that experience?

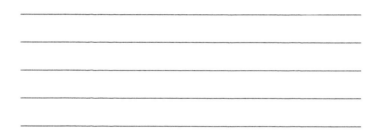

METAPHORIC SUGGESTION

A metaphoric suggestion should represent the essence of your issue. Be creative, explore, try on new images and energies. Let your creative inner mind help you to come up with good icons to use as focal points. Let these be powerful representations that speak to you and teach you.

What kind of metaphor would best characterize the energy or qualities you want to bring to your manifestation process? Describe the metaphor and what you might learn from it.

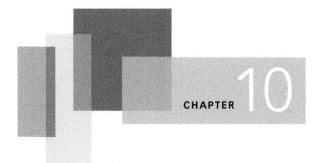

CHAPTER 10

Practice Notes

Jot down your experiences and insights from trying the various types of hypnotic suggestions. What worked best for you?

taking action—
concluding

When you are ready to complete a hypnosis session, it is useful to do a proper conclusion. It is like signing your name on a letter or saying good-bye to a friend. This is an important part of the ritual. The self-hypnosis session is now concluding. You are preparing to get up out of your comfortable chair by the fireplace to leave the house, and return to the world ready for another amazing day.

Concluding Your Session

The basic elements of the conclusion of the session are to undo any hypnotic phenomena you may have suggested, to give yourself any appropriate posthypnotic suggestions, to do a final reinforcement of the main goals of the session, to encourage a positive expectancy for future sessions, and to suggest that you will come back ready for a wonderful day, or if it is nighttime, ready for a deep sleep.

HYPNOTIC PHENOMENA

If you have used hypnotic phenomena, such as catalepsy, you will want to give yourself the suggestion that everything now returns to normal, better than normal. If, for example, you had made your hands immovable, you would suggest that they are now able to move freely and that they feel better than ever.

POSTHYPNOTIC SUGGESTION

As mentioned in chapter 8, you may want to give yourself a suggestion

PART THREE

self-hypnosis in
DAILY LIFE

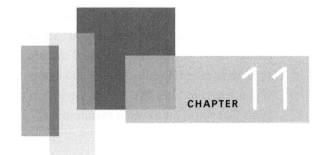

CHAPTER 11

integrating the elements

In this chapter all the pieces come together. You will be provided with a template to use to begin doing your own integrated self-hypnosis practice. You can embellish this template with ideas from earlier chapters and tailor it to suit your own preferences. Experiment and find what works best for you. In the beginning of your practice it is helpful to use a more standardized approach for a while, such as the one provided here. That will allow your mind and body to become accustomed to working with the various aspects of the hypnotic process. It also builds a sense of familiarity with the steps of self-hypnosis. If you drive the same route every day, it becomes easier to remember the way to your destination. Having a consistent and familiar method will help you to go into hypnosis more effectively.

The Goal

As described in chapter 6, having a clear sense of your desired outcomes is important. A vague goal will generate less insight, less commitment, and less motivation than a refined one. Water becomes a powerful force when it is focused and directed through a channel. Give direction to your dream, and it too will become empowering. You can also use hypnosis to arrive at a clearer vision if your issues are still muddy. Finding clarity can become your goal. Take a bit of time now and complete the exercises in chapter 6 if you have not already done so. Decide on the most important goal or goals that you want to begin manifesting.

Preparing Your Suggestions

Think of the suggestions you will want to use during your session. Make them appropriate, sufficient, positive, and varied. You will need a clear set of suggestions before you can do effective self-hypnosis. Work on the phrasing for your verbal suggestions, the imagery for your visual suggestions, and your choice of metaphors. See chapter 9 for more details about hypnotic suggestions. If you have not yet done so, work through the exercises in chapter 9 and create a set of specific verbal, visual, and metaphoric suggestions to work with.

The Setting

As mentioned in chapter 5, ideally you want to do your sessions in a setting that is conducive to relaxation, comfortable, reasonably quiet, and free from disturbances. If the lights can be lowered and some relaxing music turned on that is great. Reduce external input as much as possible, so there is less stimuli to pull your mind back out into the world. You want to create a sense of safety, relaxation, and comfort whenever possible.

Induction

Choose your induction method. In chapter 7 a variety of methods were presented for you to experiment with. The Fused Eyelids method is a good one to start with if you have not selected another one already. It is simple and very effective for most people. Whichever induction method you choose, remember that this is not about trying or struggling; it's about being and letting it flow.

Relaxation and Deepening

You can do self-hypnosis anywhere, but ideally you should find a good chair or couch to lie on. Make sure you stay warm too; use a blanket if you need it. Be comfortable. You will remember from chapter 8 that the magic words for relaxation are "warm, heavy, and relaxed." Tell yourself over and over, "I feel warm, heavy, and relaxed." That formula is simple and effective. For deepening you can use visual imagery, counting down, direct suggestion, and hypnotic phenomena. They can be used individually or in creative combinations. Counting down is a very effective approach. See chapter 8 for details.

Transformation

During your session, give your hypnotic suggestions—verbal, visual, and metaphoric. Alternate your suggestions with relaxation and other deepening methods. Continue to weave these elements to stay in the learning state while giving yourself your suggestions. See your outcome, feel it, tell yourself that you will achieve your goal, believe it. This is how old belief structures begin to dissolve and new powerful beliefs take root. Open the powerful mind-body matrix and drop in transforming images and ideas.

Conclusion

Come back. Tell yourself, "I am returning now feeling refreshed, relaxed, and ready for the day. Come back slowly, noticing your breathing and your relaxation. Undo all hypnotic phenomena. Give yourself the posthypnotic suggestion that each session will be even more effective, and that during the day the positive effects of the session will become more and more evident. You can also give a posthypnotic trigger that will help you to reactivate the desired thought or behavior you are seeking to manifest.

Summary of Steps

- Vision your priority goals for greatest success and happiness
- Focus with your breath and induction
- Deepen with relaxation and other deepening methods
- Transform with verbal, visual, and metaphoric suggestions
- Cycle—for as long as you have time, cycle through your relaxation deepening methods and suggestions over and over to help you stay in a suitable state for deep transformation to occur)
- Conclude the process, coming back slowly, ready for the day

Sample Script

This book is designed in a modular fashion, providing the elements needed to sequentially build an effective self-hypnosis session. In each of the previous chapters many ideas were presented for you to explore, to see what works best for you. Rather than just providing prefabricated recipes, a one-size-fits-all approach, the elements of self-hypnosis were explained, so that you could ultimately create more finely tuned, personalized approaches. Because of this modular approach you can mix and match ideas from the various chapters as you see fit. In addition, the next chapter has many ideas for working with specific issues that provide useful material to include in your session.

The following script is built from the elements of each chapter. It is offered both as an example and also as a useful framework for doing your own self-hypnosis sessions. It can be a good starting point, and as you become more familiar and comfortable with the material in the book you can bring in other methods and modify the script. If you choose to use this sample framework then read it to yourself several times to get a sense of the integrated process. As soon as possible, put the script down and just paraphrase the concepts in your mind. If you like you can also make a tape for yourself. It is easy to do, and it can be a useful way to work with your goals. You can write a short script, incorporating some of the ideas on specific issues from the next chapter, fine-tune the message, and then record it. The whole process will probably take an hour or two. You will then have a tailored product for your transformational process. If you do record your script then it can be a good idea to change the words "I and my" to "You and your." In this way the recording has the quality of someone speaking to you, which has a more engaging effect.

So give it a go. The core script provided here includes the following elements to work with:

- **Focusing.**

- **Fused Eyelids Induction.**

- **Relaxation and Deepening** including direct suggestions, counting down, floating leaf imagery, the hypnotic phenomena of catalepsy (immovable legs), and special workplace imagery.

- **Suggestions** focusing on the specific topic of self-confidence for its verbal, visual, and metaphoric suggestion content. (As you create your own scripts it always useful to include core themes of self-confidence, the capacity to love, and a sense of having a deeply meaningful life.)

- **Concluding** with the posthypnotic suggestion of confidence during day before we undo the hypnotic phenomena.

So let us begin. Find a quiet, relaxing spot. Put on some peaceful music. Turn the lights down. Loosen any tight clothes, take off glasses and shoes. If you have to be finished by a certain time or if you are concerned that you might fall asleep, set a quiet alarm. Sit or lie down. Cover yourself with a blanket if desired. Get comfortable and gently gaze into the space in front of you.

FOCUSING

I will now take three deep breaths. [Take three slow, deep breaths.] Each breath allows me to let go and to begin relaxing. Three deep, relaxing breaths. Each breath out allows my muscles to soften, to become more comfortable. It feels so good to take this time for myself, time to manifest my vision, my life dreams. I know my dreams will come true. I know that everything I experience, every sound, every thought, every feeling and sensation will help me to go even deeper inside, into a place of safety, a place of comfort, a place of deep transformation. I continue to notice my body and mind relaxing. My breath is quieting. Every exhale helps me to relax even more deeply, more completely. I feel the chair/couch/bed beneath me, totally supporting me, completely supporting my body. It lets me relax completely. Letting go of every muscle now. Completely relaxing. My face, shoulders, arms, legs, breath, mind are so comfortably relaxed. I let go of every muscle now.

FUSED EYELIDS INDUCTION

As I continue to relax I notice that my eyelids are becoming heavier and heavier. They are wonderfully heavy, just wanting to close. I know that when they do close I will go even deeper inside. My eyelids are getting heavier and heavier, so heavy, so relaxed. They just want to close to take me deep inside, into that place where dreams become real. My entire body is getting more heavy, more relaxed. Warm currents of comforting energy are flowing through me, just flowing through me. The colors are so beautiful. It is a perfect temperature. My eyelids are getting so heavy, taking me deeper and deeper inside. When they close I will not be able to open them. They will be so incredibly heavy. They will not open until my session is done, or until I am ready to open them. They are getting incredibly heavy, incredibly relaxed. Taking me deeper and deeper inside. [Repeat until eyes close.]

RELAXATION AND DEEPENING

My legs and arms are warm, heavy, and relaxed. I am floating in warm water, just floating. It feels so wonderful. [Repeat these phrases several times.] Slowly I begin sinking down, sinking down into a warm ocean of energy. With each exhalation I am going deeper and deeper inside. It is a very comforting feeling, very relaxing. Twenty. I am floating down now. Nineteen. Like a leaf floating down toward the earth. Feeling more and more wonderfully relaxed, more and more comfortable. Eighteen. My mind and body are going deeper, floating down. Seventeen. With every exhale I go deeper and deeper inside. The forest is quiet, peaceful. Sixteen. Everything is letting go. Floating slowly down toward the earth, just letting go and floating. Fifteen. As I float down I am aware of a sense of deep peace. Fourteen. My body and mind are floating down deeper and deeper. The earth gently pulls me with its vast healing energy. Thirteen. My legs feel immovable; they are becoming so heavy and relaxed. My legs feel immovable; they are becoming so heavy and relaxed. Twelve. I am floating down. Eleven. I feel incredibly heavy, wonderfully heavy. Such an amazing feeling. Floating down toward the earth. Ten. Sinking deeper and deeper into the energy beneath me. Nine. Body and mind are melting into this peaceful space, very peaceful, very spacious. Beautiful colors, feeling so comfortable. Eight. It feels so relaxing. Deeper. Like an ocean, underwater canyons, deep. Seven. Deeper and deeper inside. Six. My legs are immovable. They are so heavy. The heavier they become the deeper inside I go. Five. Slowly floating in a vast spiral of energy, deeper and deeper, on warm currents of light. They are so heavy. The heavier they become the deeper I go inside. Deeper down, floating. Four. Floating deeper and deeper. Three. The colors are calming, so soothing, calming, so soothing. It is so peaceful here. Two. I am sinking deeper and deeper toward a beautiful light. One. I enter that light deep beneath me. Floating down into the light. Dissolving, just dissolving into that peaceful light.

WORKPLACE IMAGERY

I am in a most amazing place now, an incredible grotto. There is a small waterfall and a crystal pool of sparkling water. There is a perfect place for me to lie down on the smooth, warm rocks, like nature's reclining chair. It fits my body perfectly. It is so comfortable, completely supporting my body. It is incredibly comfortable. As I sit there a leopard comes and lies down in front of me. I feel its weight pressing against my feet. I recognize this to be a guardian animal of this place, here to protect me. Floating on the surface of the pond is a beautiful pulsing light, an orb like a small radiant star. Directly beyond that is the waterfall. As I look at the waterfall its warm, translucent waters appear to display images. I can see images of my life. My body and mind are transfixed, immovable, so deeply relaxed. The air is fresh with the scent of pine and some incredible energy. It fills my body, and I can feel a healing energy, a purifying light, going into every cell. It fills every thought, every memory, every dream. The grotto is surrounded by ancient trees that rise up endlessly to the blue sky above. The rock wall surfaces are smooth and rounded. Moist ferns cover one wall. I watch the waters flowing and listen to the sounds.

VERBAL SUGGESTION

I feel power running through my body and mind. I feel incredible. My energy is pure light. I remember who I am, where I am from, why I am here, how precious this adventure of life truly is. I have a wonderful sense that I can do anything at all, whatever I set my mind to. I believe in myself. I know what I can do, how many things are possible once I make my commitment to change, to grow, to heal, to succeed. I am committed now. The world needs me to be my fullest self. The world needs me to be my fullest self. The world needs me. I am alive now. I feel incredible. [Insert specific personalized suggestions.]

_____

_____

VISUAL SUGGESTION

I can see colors from behind the waterfall, like large shining gems. I see the color red, like some amazing ruby light. It is pure, extremely beautiful, very powerful, very intense. This light is flowing in a beam toward me, filling me with power like the morning sun. I am standing on a beautiful beach watching the sun rising up over the pure ocean. I see myself looking grateful, arms stretching up toward the sky. I am floating. I am powerful, so relaxed, so comfortable. It has been a most incredible year. I have done more, felt better, been stronger, kinder, more patient and persistent than at any time in my life. I look amazed and delighted. I see myself filled with confidence, the power of believing that I can. As I turn around I see down the beach my wiser, older self, twenty years into the future. A wiser, older self who has lived a powerful, self-respecting, confident life. I see a self that is capable, kind, courageous, powerful, very alive. That self sends a message that I feel deep inside. [Visualize any specific desired outcomes as completely as possible. Bring in positive emotion.]

METAPHORIC SUGGESTION

As I sit here I sense the energy of my leopard guardian. I sense the leopard within me, the courage, the intensity, the sheer power. I feel the freedom of life, the power of life deep within my own roots. I am alive now. [Select appropriate metaphoric symbol.]

RELAXATION, DEEPENING, AND SUGGESTIONS

[Repeat this cycle until finished.] I hear a voice from the light star floating on the pool. It tells me to close my eyes. I continue to go deeper and deeper inside. I feel so incredibly comfortable and relaxed. My mind and body are so comfortable, such a beautiful color, such a comfortable feeling. Like floating down toward the earth. The more relaxed I become the deeper inside I go, deeper into confidence, deeper into power, deeper into self-respect. I see myself waking up in the morning with an inspiration. I am empowered by an incredible energy throughout the day that helps me to accomplish everything I need to do to move closer to my dreams. I feel incredible, warm, comfortable, relaxed. I am going deeper and deeper inside with each exhale. Like a leaf floating down deeper toward the power, deeper into an ocean of energy. Dissolving. Each exhale takes me deeper into this comfort, into this relaxation, deeper into confident peace. I can see my leopard body. I am stretching, claws digging into the side of a tree. My body is strong, supple, energetic, powerful. I sit quietly, watching, unstirred, powerful. I feel incredibly confident. I know I can do whatever I need to do to reach my dreams. I believe. Every exhalation takes me deeper and deeper into relaxation. During the week, every day at noon I will remember the sun in the sky above, and I will feel a surge of confidence. I will feel the ruby red energy of life filling me with confidence. I am filled with light and energy. I feel incredible. When I see the red color of a stop sign, I will stop. I will feel the power. I will be filled with a sense of pure confidence and joy, grateful to be alive. I love my life. I love life. I love life. I believe in life. I believe in myself. Life helps me in so many ways. Life is great. People are wonderful. I love my life.

CONCLUDING

My dreams will come to me. I can see my goal totally, clearly. I will take a moment to let this experience integrate into my understanding deeply. I take a deep breath and let the images and ideas of success go deep inside me. Taking a breath I inhale these images, feelings, insights deep into myself. I see myself looking very accomplished, very happy. I know that whatever is perfect and best for me will come to pass. I notice my body now, my breathing. My eyelids feel normal, comfortable and refreshed. My eyelids feel perfect. My legs feel perfect, strong and relaxed. My legs feel wonderful. I am coming back feeling refreshed, relaxed, and ready for life. Each of my sessions will be more and more effective. This is going to be the most amazing week of my life. I feel incredible, and I anticipate positive success all week long. I come back slowly now, feeling great. Whenever I am ready, I slowly open my eyes to a most amazing day.

Short Version

Close your eyes, take several deep breaths, relax. Count down from twenty to one. During the counting down, tell yourself that you are feeling warm, heavy, and relaxed and that you are going deeper and deeper inside. You can imagine walking down a set of beautiful stairs or down a path. When you reach the number one, see yourself in a very beautiful, safe place, such as under a palm tree on a perfect beach.

Relax there for a moment.

Introduce suggestion: tell yourself about your success; see your outcome imagery; bring in a metaphoric symbol that supports your outcome vision. Give yourself a posthypnotic suggestion to reactivate positive expectation during the day.

Come back feeling refreshed, relaxed, and peaceful.

Priming

One other very useful quick strategy is an approach I call priming. This method can be used as a simple method to prepare for each day. Done early in the morning it sets the tone for everything you will do. It can also be done right before specific important events to give an increased sense of power and positive expectancy of achieving desired outcomes. The following version is used to prime the entire day. It is done in the morning before the day begins. To do priming just follow these eight simple steps:

1. Close your eyes and relax.

2. See yourself at the end of the day. You are sitting in a comfortable chair in your home. You look very happy, like you have had one of the most incredible days of your life so far.

3. Tell yourself mentally why it has been such an incredible day. Tell yourself that you successfully met your objectives for the specific things that you had to do for the day. For example, in my priming I might tell myself that I had an incredible day at work, extremely productive, that I was positive and supportive of people I met, that I worked out and my body feels great, that I ate healthy food. Pick a few of the key things for the day, your top daily or general life goals.

4. As you describe these things visualize them to the extent possible.

5. Bring positive feeling into the visual images (on certain days this may require a bit of effort).

6. Tell yourself that you feel incredible, that it has been one of the most amazing days of your life so far.

7. When you feel complete, inhale this energy deep into the center of your being, and then exhale it out into the universe.

8. Slowly open your eyes and begin your most amazing day.

To prime specific events, use the basic eight step process. Instead of seeing yourself at the end of the day, however, see yourself at the end of the specific event. See yourself as successful, happy, enthused, and specify that you are happy because of the positive nature of the event. Priming can be done for microevents, such as preparing to make an important phone call, all the way to macroevents, such as priming the day, month, or year.

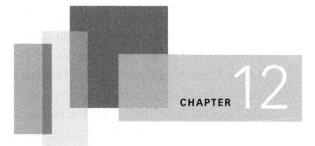

specific applications

In the previous chapters we have been building a format for doing self-hypnotic work. Now that all the elements are in place you can begin working with issues of personal interest. This chapter presents a broad range of issues and provides useful ideas for beginning your own self-hypnosis practice. If your particular goal area is not found here then select a related topic and work with the ideas provided. The following topics are presented:

- Addiction and habit control
- Anxiety, phobia, fear, stress
- Body image
- Career
- Childbirth
- Emotions and attitudes
- Energy
- Financial security and prosperity
- Health and healing
- Insomnia
- Learning

- Pain
- Procrastination
- Relationships and love
- Sales and business
- Self-confidence, shyness, self-love
- Sexual health
- Skin conditions
- Sports and performance
- Weight management

Each topic in this chapter is approached comprehensively with the intention of providing ideas to begin creating an effective self-hypnosis transformation process. Under each one you will find three sections: Action Layers, Hypnotic Suggestions, and Personal Plans. In the Action Layers, ideas are given for addressing the personal, behavioral, or environmental aspects of the issue. The Person layer focuses on a balanced body, calm and positive emotions, and a focused mind. The Behavior layer gives ideas for constructive, empowered action. The Environment layer examines how to make the external world support your success. The Hypnotic Suggestions include ideas for creating purposeful and effective verbal, visual, and metaphoric suggestions. Verbal suggestions should be positive and personal and have present and future perspectives. They should state clearly and strongly exactly what you want to hear so you will feel encouraged and capable. Visual suggestions should present as clear a picture as possible of what you truly want your life to look like. Metaphoric suggestions are best if they are strong, clear iconic images that empower you to succeed. Each topic concludes with a Personal Plans section where you can develop specific steps for beginning to make your own transformational process a reality. Take some time now to work with the following topics. Find your topic, work with the action layers and suggestions, add additional ideas from other resources such as issue-relevant books or websites, and create a tailored package for your success.

Addiction and Habit Control

ACTION LAYERS

Person

Dealing effectively with addiction involves working with emotional obstacles, challenging thoughts, and physical discomfort. Underlying emotional issues can be difficult to isolate, understand, and modify. They may be experienced as fear, unworthiness, helplessness, survival concerns, or a desire to die. You will need to develop a stronger sense of self-worth, positiveness, and a belief in your own abilities. You will also want to develop your ability to relax deeply and let go of tension, learning to use relaxation to work with physical discomfort and uneasiness. The key is to get your body and mind balanced again and to activate the power stay in balance.

Be patient, love yourself, and be proud of yourself for doing the work. Do not give up. Know that you can do it.

Behavior

Addiction and habits can relate to drugs, alcohol, tobacco, food, gambling, nail biting, shopping, and other behaviors. A key to changing any of them is to pay attention to the addictive pattern—when, where, why, and how much. When you start self-monitoring your pattern in this way you make it more conscious. So pay close attention to the pattern. This helps awaken the change process. Once you recognize the pattern you can start to do it differently, to break up the automatic behaviors. For example, you can change the time when you do it; you can do the steps of the pattern in a different order or change the speed, the location, or who you do them with; or do whatever you can think of to break up the habitual pattern. This helps some people change behaviors. Find new ways to make life work.

Environment

You may need to change elements of your environment to succeed in becoming independent. If you associate with other people who are struggling with their own addiction, they will challenge your success. Most likely, you will need to make new friends. That can be hard, but we are talking about your life. You will also need to regulate your environment to keep away from the thing that you are addicted to. Keep it out of your home, and avoid people and places where you can easily obtain it. Ask for help. Join a support group. There are many 12-step programs and other resources around that can be useful.

HYPNOTIC SUGGESTIONS

Verbal

I know I will survive. I know I am safe. I love myself and seek out others who respect themselves and who respect me. I am capable, and I am learning new ways to make my life work better and better. I deserve to live. I deal with any urges easily and effectively because I am strong. I enjoy my life free of _____. I am balanced and healthy, and I only do those things that bring me true happiness, strength, peace, and balance. I associate with people who are healthy and strong. I go to places that are life supportive and avoid those that are not. The old habit was about not loving myself. I love myself now, and that is why the habit is gone. I love who I am.

Visual Imagery

See yourself as addiction free. See yourself as dealing with urges very effectively now and being free of any urges. Imagine a relaxed, happy, confident you. You look great. See yourself one year and five years out in the future being independent, healthy, and very happy.

Metaphoric

Find an image that triggers a specific feeling that helps you deal with this change. For example, if you need to feel strong you could use an image of a brick wall (immovable in your commitment to finally loving yourself.) Maybe the word *love* is written on that wall. If you need courage you could use an image of a lion. Become the powerful lion. Feel the natural power within yourself. You could imagine a wise person who can offer you counsel. Ask them what they think you should do.

PERSONAL PLANS

Anxiety, Phobia, Fear, and Stress

ACTION LAYERS

Person

Relaxation is very, very helpful. Get your body vibrating at a lower, quieter level. Practice some relaxation method before a stressful event, such as right before an exam starts or right before a performance. Try a one minute method or priming. Banish any fearful thoughts, just banish them. Make them leave. You can also turn the fear into a small brother or sister. Take it by the hand and walk with it, but do not let it run and drag you. Talk to that small frightened child and reassure him or her. Remember, it is the vulnerable aspect of self that is afraid. Also focus on your goal and feel your passion. This makes obstacles smaller or invisible. Go with your passion. You have a purpose to fulfill. Focus on your goal, where you are going. Also, very important, remember to breathe deeply and slowly when you are anxious. Inhale through your nostrils. Breathe down into your abdomen. Exhale slowly.

Behavior

Reduce behaviors that increase your anxiety, such as procrastination and being late, alienating people because of your social fear, or drinking caffeinated beverages. Manage time, say no, get clear on your goals, and be responsible. You will succeed. Laugh, smile, do fun things, learn to be more at ease with things, get out of your head, go for walks at the beach, listen to quieting music, reduce your use of drugs and alcohol and stimulants such as coffee, keep your life in order, make more positive friends. Learn to meditate.

Environment

Reduce the number of things in your environment that increase your stress, such as angry people, stressful work, excess noise, clutter, and other imbalancing stimuli. Create a peaceful space. It can be helpful to use resources in the environment that can soothe the energy body, such as homeopathy and herbal products.

HYPNOTIC SUGGESTIONS

Verbal

I am calm and relaxed. My body is warm, heavy, and relaxed. I move toward my goals steadily. My mind is peaceful. Fear and negative thoughts flow out of me with each exhale. I am left clear and filled with happiness. I feel more and more relaxed every day. I am strong and confident; I manage my time and space. My life is organized and balanced. I make choices in my life that increase my sense of calm and peace. Relaxation is one of my main goals. I look forward to each day and to the opportunity to learn from life. I am flexible, happy, resourceful, and strong. I feel fantastic.

Visual Imagery

See yourself as being very calm and relaxed. Imagine being in a hot tub, in a cabin in the woods, or sitting on a sandy beach. When stress-inducing images come to mind during the day, modify them, make the images small and insignificant. Banish them; you are powerful. You have incredible power over them and with practice that power will grow. Take the reigns, change negative patterns, and substitute positive images for every negative one. Whatever your fear image is, during self-hypnosis see the opposite.

Metaphoric

Be a mighty warrior or champion fighter. Experience yourself interacting with all things with confidence. Use this as a metaphor of immense power. Or be like a child learning, playing, and having fun with life. Or be like a wise person who knows a great deal about life and is quite capable at dealing with events as they flow by. The old sage sits by the river of life and wisely observes the flow of life. All things come to that wise being in time. Be that sage.

Other Ideas

With phobia we often find a clear interrelationship between: person (negative imagery, internal feelings of fear, and physical discomfort); behavior (avoidance); and environment (fear-evoking stimuli). One of the easiest ways to work with this trinity is to disrupt it at one of its three points. A very effective method is to experience a deep state of relaxation (opposite of body discomfort) when you encounter the anxiety-provoking item.

To do this, work on creating very deep relaxation. Give yourself the suggestion that you will feel that relaxing energy whenever you come across the evocative stimuli. This will begin to create a new pattern, disrupting the old pattern of stimuli, fear, and avoidance. Be patient with the fear and with yourself, and you will transform.

PERSONAL PLANS

Body Image

ACTION LAYERS

Person

Deal with negative thoughts and internal criticism. It is a very useful exercise to take a one-day or a one-week break from self-criticism. That can be a very challenging process but very insight producing. It oftens lets us see how damaging and constant the barrage of our negative internal dialogue can be. Once apparent, it can become quite motivating to do something about that aspect of our mind, such as using self-hypnosis to reduce this critical voice, making it tiny, weak, and faint. Get an image of the voice's source and play with that image.

It is important to reduce negative feelings about yourself and bring in more happiness. Start thinking in more positive ways about yourself. Consciously use inner praise. Create some simple, positive affirmations and put them to regular use. No one says this is easy to do, but it is a necessary task. Practice being happy and loving yourself. Ultimately it does not matter how big or how small those unappreciated body parts are. It is the person inside your body, your accepting self, that will be the ultimate source of your happiness.

Behavior

Avoid behaviors that are self-destructive or harmful to your body. Your healing will require self-love and avoiding behaviors that are not self loving. The neurotic mind can make certain behaviors appear okay, but if they cause you pain in any way they are not okay. Take good care of your body, exercise, eat nutritious food, rest, spend time with people you care about, meditate, play. Developing a strong and healthy body will help you to feel good regardless of whether or not you fit some cultural body norm. Exercise is great medicine for the mind and the body.

Environment

Associate with people who love you for who you are. Get rid of critics. Throw away the glamour and body building magazines. Listen to your body and what is good for it, not some cultural hallucination of what a body should look like. If your body image issues are causing depression or other problems that are significantly bothersome then you might want to seek professional help or at least to join a support group to see that you are not alone and to get ideas of what you can do to feel better about your life and yourself.

HYPNOTIC SUGGESTIONS

Verbal

I love myself for who I am. I am a wonderful person, and I love my body completely. My body is my friend, and I am its caretaker. I love every part of myself. I am taking care of my body. I am exercising and eating well and getting rest. My life is balanced, and I have a positive attitude about life. I look forward to getting up every morning and living each day to the fullest. There are so many people in this world who have so little. I am a very fortunate person and am grateful to be here now. I love who I am, and I am feeling more and more confidence and self-love every day.

Visual Imagery

See yourself looking in a mirror at your body in a very kind and loving way. See a guardian angel talking to you and teaching you about self-love. You can also imagine your negative internal voice. Make it into an image or a color or shape. Then modify that negative voice image in ways that feel good to you. Change its color, shape, size, or location. Make the image very, very tiny. Make its voice very small, infantile. Release it and send it off into the light. Watch it dissolve and be transformed. Watch to see what becomes of that image as it is sent into the light to receive a healing.

Metaphoric

Let your body be a temple which holds a sacred energy—you, your essential energy, your Self, spirit, or life.

PERSONAL PLANS

Career

ACTION LAYERS

Person

Develop and maintain a positive belief that you will come to know what type of work you want and that you will find ideal work for yourself. Be confident; deal with doubts and fears. Be optimistic and persistent. Get out there every day. Keep your spirits up, your motivation high. If you begin to get down, if things get slow, take some time off and rest. Believe in yourself and know there is a place to put your talents to work. Another strategy is to love the job you have until you find the job you want. Be happy now.

Behavior

Go to the career section in your local public or university library and use it. Do informational interviews. Go to a community college and take their career orientation tests. Read the help wanted ads. Network and join organizations where you can get job leads. Get out there every day and knock on doors. Keep at it. Be thoughtful in your approach: plan and use your time wisely. Do not hesitate to ask people you know for ideas and connections. Follow up on your leads. Go to job fairs. Talk to recruiters. Check in the places where your type of work would be advertised. Upgrade your letterhead and business cards, any materials that represent you. Be professional in your appearance and behavior.

Environment

Go where the work is, where there is a concentration of jobs and hiring. It is hard to find water in a desert. The job you want might mean moving to a larger city or another state. Match your skills to the needs of the area you live in, or move, or get new skills. Get more technical or professional training if you need it. Like it or not, it is a job market, and we need to offer skills that people want to buy. Stay in touch with the information on marketable skills and upgrade as necessary to stay competitive.

HYPNOTIC SUGGESTIONS

Verbal

I have career clarity. I get interviews and do extremely well. People like me the moment the interview starts. I know exactly what to say. I let my skills shine. I have a great job. I love the work I am doing (say this whether you have a job or not; you can specify the ideal job here as that creates a positive mental expectancy for that job). It is perfect for me in every way. My work makes me very happy. I love my job. I am excellent at what I do. My abilities are developing daily. I am a great contributor to my workplace. We create a powerful team, and I am succeeding in this place.

Visual Imagery

For career selection: If you know what your career goal is, count down from twenty to one as you imagine yourself walking down a hallway. At the end of the hall there is a door. When you reach the number one, open the door and see yourself inside that space doing what you want to do.

For job hunting: Imagine yourself working in that job or company. See yourself signing paperwork from the company. See yourself being very productive and very happy working there.

Metaphoric

Be like a hand putting on a very well-made glove. It is a perfect fit and it feels great.

PERSONAL PLANS

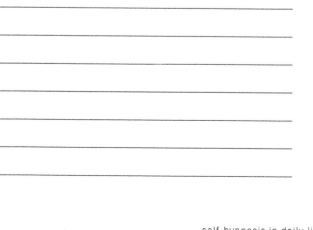

Childbirth

ACTION LAYERS

Person

Keep your body healthy. Learn to relax very deeply. Banish fear and create positive expectations. Anticipate a wonderful, enjoyable experience. Be positive. Be calm. Relax your body. Relax your mind. Relax your emotions. Use self-hypnosis to promote a healthy pregnancy, delivery, and baby. Create powerful positive expectancy on all levels.

Behavior

Work regularly with relaxation, learning how to relax the muscles of your body, how to calm your mind. Practice the deep breathing methods taught in birthing classes. Practice those methods and associate that breathing with very positive, happy feelings. Join a birthing class to learn such useful skills. Stay healthy, take your vitamins, get your exercise, enjoy the process, and think of what a truly amazing event you are participating in.

Environment

Keep your environment positive and healthy during your pregnancy. Eat well, rest, and be positive. Avoid tobacco, drugs, and alcohol. Get assistance if this is an issue. Pregnancy is an excellent time for healing old patterns and becoming a new person. Have your coach, partner, or other supportive people with you during delivery. Prepare the nest. Create a healthy, safe, loving space for your new family member.

HYPNOTIC SUGGESTIONS

You will ideally want to work on these practices for several months before the birth. Try to do some relaxation and imagery work every day.

Verbal

This is going to be a very smooth and wonderful birth. My baby is going to be healthy and happy. I will relax and breathe my baby into the world. My body feels strong and healthy during this pregnancy, and I feel very relaxed and calm during the delivery. My baby comes into this world easily, calm and incredibly healthy. I feel deep happiness during the entire process. Time passes quickly. It all goes so easily, so smoothly. I am warm, heavy, and relaxed. Once the baby arrives safe and healthy, my body will heal incredibly quickly.

Visual Imagery

See yourself having your baby easily and effortlessly. Your baby just flows out of you like light or an ocean wave, very healthy and happy. See yourself and everyone who loves you filled with joy. You are holding your baby and telling the baby how easy the birth was, how healthy, loved, and special he or she is.

Metaphoric

Here is a metaphor that is useful for delivery. Let it be spring, a nice time to hike down to the river. The waters are full. You can feel the joyful vibrations of the springtime river flowing. The waters are warm and easy, flowing effortlessly from the mountaintop to the vast blue ocean. The river feels its happiness and your happiness. It is a warm and joyful water moving down the mountain slope. Be joyful too.

PERSONAL PLANS

Emotions and Attitudes

ACTION LAYERS

Person

Work on finding, creating, and installing positive attitudes and emotions. It is not easy to feel good if you are depressed or sad, so you will need to take some action to pull out of that state. Remove self-criticism from your mind, if only for one day or one hour at a time. This one-day fast from negativity will help to retrain your mind. Find your goals, focus on them, believe in yourself. All successful people believe in themselves. You do too. Have faith in the perfection of all things.

Behavior

Do something. Have more fun, meet people, do your work and love it, praise all things. Say yes to life. Physical activity and exercise can lighten and help generate more positive emotions. Find the things that make you happy—funny movies, uplifting music—do what you need to do to shift your state toward the positive. Eat right and avoid excess alcohol, which is a mild depressant. Also avoid excess sugars and fats. Get plenty of rest.

Environment

Stay with a positive crowd. Avoid the complainers. As one of my favorite bumper stickers says, "Look for the good and praise it." Look for things around you to be happy about. Help others to see the good around you too. Show them the rainbow or the flowers in the sidewalk. Find as many things in your life as you can to be grateful for.

HYPNOTIC SUGGESTIONS

Verbal

I work productively with my emotions. I honor my feelings. My emotions are in balance. I have a powerful, positive attitude. I take responsibility for my success. I love my goals, and my actions are powerful. My life will change this world in a positive way. I love my life. I love this world.

Visual

See yourself as happy, having fun. See your surroundings as encouraging and positive. Imagine yourself walking down the street and people congratulating you on your good work and success. You can see a large radiant energy around your body. It is a wonderful color. It makes you feel great. You condense this energy down to a small sphere, the size of a small stone. You put it in your mouth and swallow it. That light energy is in you so you can access it at any time. You can expand it at any time, and when you are done shrink it down and swallow it again. That powerful energy is always with you. See yourself doing something that you have done or could imagine doing that would be extremely energizing. Be in that image.

Metaphoric

Be a winged horse soaring high into the light of the sun. Imagine that you are a powerful person, like a king or queen, a high priestess, or a warrior. Feel that energy; be that person.

PERSONAL PLANS

Energy

ACTION LAYERS

Person

Develop a positive mental attitude. Give yourself inspirational talks. Imagine that people are applauding you, like you are crossing the finish line, a winner. Energize yourself mentally. In the morning sing yourself an "I feel great" song to build your positive energy for the day. Remember that you are a learner. You are learning what you need to know to be happy. Remind yourself over and over that you will succeed, that you can do it. Self-love is also very energizing. Remove the garbage about yourself and your world from your mind. Just throw it out.

Behavior

Eat right. Enjoy the foods that make you feel light, happy, clear minded and able to work. Avoid excess in eating; it is hard on the digestive system. Stop smoking completely. Reduce use of unnecessary drugs. Also reduce alcohol consumption as it is a mild depressant. Exercise will increase general well-being and energy. Keep your life balanced. Discipline yourself, in a positive way. Place your goals out where you can see them to remind you of what you want in life. Track them and reward yourself for every success. The clearer and more committed and more enthusiastic you are about your dream, the more energy you will possess. Read about passionate people like Thomas Edison or John Muir. Passion is very energizing, and your dream is a strong connection to your passion. Live a life of no regrets. Go for your dream. Create your own joyful, energizing song and sing it in the shower each morning.

Environment

Get the junk food out of your house. Make it easy to exercise—buy a jump rope, move closer to the park, whatever will help. Keep images around the house, such as magazines that display active, energetic people.

HYPNOTIC SUGGESTIONS

Verbal

I am powerful, alive, and dynamic. Energy flows through me. I feel great. I feel incredible. I love my life. I am powerful, productive, organized, energetic, and totally effective. I can feel the power of life flowing through me. I feel the power of the earth, the sky, the wind, the water, the sun. The goodness of the world is in my heart and mind, and that power lifts me higher. I am strong and healthy. The radiant power of the sun is warming me. The surging power of the ocean is moving me. I am a warrior.

Visual

See yourself looking completely excited about life. You look very happy and enthusiastic. Perhaps you are jumping up and down with your arms up in the air shouting, "Yes." See yourself energized and feeling the power of life. See yourself doing something that totally energizes you—something physical, making a great deal, completing a major project. Get into a memory of personal power.

Metaphoric

Become an animal that represents full personal energy for you. You could become a galloping wild horse or a lion. Become something powerful and feel that power within you.

PERSONAL PLANS

Financial Security and Prosperity

ACTION LAYERS

Person

Money is a mental symbol. What does money symbolize for you—freedom, safety, abundance? Remember to consider your deepest values. If freedom is your core value and you gain a lot of money but not freedom, where are you? Money is a practical resource. Acquire it and use it wisely. It is important that you now strongly embrace the belief that it is easy for you to make money.

Behavior

Set some financial goals for a year, five years, and your lifetime. How much do you want to be worth five years from now, twenty years? Get reading materials on money management and investing. There is a lot of good material out there; become informed. Remember, it is easier to be wealthy by living simply than it is by trying to make enough to live extravagantly. Be a pragmatic consumer. Do not be manipulated by consumption consciousness; spend wisely. Earn, save, invest. Ask your inner mind for help and ideas. Think in the long term.

Environment

Find someone that you know or that you see on the news, who represents financial success for you. Emulate that person, become him or her, think like that successful figure. Pretend that you know how they think. It works. Put up images of your dream home, retirement images of being on a sandy beach, things that motivate you to save and invest for the future. Put the images where you will see them periodically.

HYPNOTIC SUGGESTIONS

Verbal

I am abundant; money flows into my life. I am grateful for what I have. My success will benefit the entire world. The universe supports my success. I deserve to be abundant in every way. The path to financial success welcomes me and supports me.

Visual

Imagine yourself on a television program being interviewed as a very successful business person (or related success imagery). See an image of yourself in your desired outcome state. See yourself having the house, car, and friends that you will have. See it clearly.

Metaphoric

Be the ocean. Many streams and rivers run down into the ocean. The ocean gathers and manages those resources well. The ocean also continually relinquishes water in the form of rain to benefit the land masses and life forms, knowing that more water will always return enriched with soil and nutrients. It is a powerful win-win model that works very effectively. Be like an arrow moving to your target. You are flying fast and direct. Nothing can stop you until you reach your goal.

PERSONAL PLANS

Health and Healing

Person

A positive attitude and a positive belief are very important. Hold strongly in your mind that you will be healthy and whole. Allow your mind to work constantly on bringing more strength to your body. Every thought, negative or positive, produces some effect. Seek to increase the number of positive thoughts moving through you and reducing the number of negative thoughts. Regulate your emotions, keep them smooth. Be positive and optimistic; deal with depression, anger, and other emotions that may burden you. If your emotions become imbalanced use creative measures, such as brief self-hypnosis, to return to center. Keep your body energy balanced.

Behavior

Do things that make you happy, bring you energy, help you remain optimistic, heal you. Eat right. Food is the first medicine in many ancient systems. One of the simplest ways to eat well is to eat for nutrients rather than caloric content. If you eat for nutrients you will be eating food that provides energy. Also, a light diet, one that is easy to digest, is good for healing. In ancient China they would cook rice soups for many, many hours to make them easy to assimilate for people who were ill. Eat foods that nourish deeply. Eat local, organic, and natural. Avoid pesticides and genetically modified foods. Eat what nature intended, not what the corporations mandate. Do what you need to do to get well. Be positive and proactive. Exercise appropriately if possible. Movement is good medicine. Walk, swim, ride a bike, stretch gently, whatever you can manage. Get fresh air when possible. Drink clean water.

Environment

Associate with positive people. Stay in healing energy places. Bring healing energy into your environment, such as plants, positive pictures and books, light, and fresh air. Get outside. Be in nature. Reduce the pollutants, energy emissions, toxic chemicals, and molds in your home and workplace if possible. Avoid toxic places, people, and things.

HYPNOTIC SUGGESTIONS
Verbal
I am getting stronger and healthier. Healing energy is flowing into my body from a very powerful place in the universe. I feel strong and whole. The universal life force is moving through me. Healing energy is flowing into me now. That energy is filling me with light, with freshness, with vitality. All toxic, stagnant energy is being removed from me. I am filled with light. Each cell of my body is glowing. I feel great. My body is a powerhouse. I am like a new plant. My leaves are catching the rays of the sun, and my body is creating energy. I am totally alive and feel powerful. I rest so deeply when I close my eyes. Each breath heals me. I am rested, healed, happy, alive.

Visual
See yourself as energetic, whole, and happy. Send healing energy (pick a powerful healing color) to any part of your mind and body that needs healing. Send healing sounds, words, or phrases to those areas; make them up, let them come from your deep mind. Let your deep mind guide you to take right action. Feel healing energy flowing through you, like an energy stream. Imagine that there is a powerful being, like a healing angel, working on you. Receive the healing. See yourself breathing in good, healing chi or energy and exhaling toxic, stagnant, putrid energy. Each breath heals you, energizes you.

Metaphoric
When you toss a stone into a pond it sinks, disappearing from sight, and the surface soon becomes calm again. Let your illness be that stone making momentary ripples, then sinking and disappearing. Let your entire energy field become balanced and harmonious again. Let your energy become smooth and calm. Imagine yourself as a radiant being, having a body of pure light.

PERSONAL PLANS

_____

_____

_____

_____

_____

_____

_____

_____

_____

_____

_____

_____

_____

_____

Insomnia

ACTION LAYERS

Person

Learn to relax. Do a lot of relaxation practice—feel warm, heavy, and relaxed. When in bed focus on your body instead of on your thoughts and feelings. When your mind starts rolling away on some idea, bring it back into your body, focusing on warm, heavy, and relaxed body feelings. Relax your body from your toes to your ears. When you are ready to sleep, then stop thinking about things. Successful people leave their work at work. Sleep is your time. Use it to heal. A good night's sleep will help you deal better with everything when you wake up. Let it go.

Behavior

Try the counting down method with the words warm, heavy, and relaxed. Count down from one hundred to one, telling yourself that you feel more comfortable with each number down. Before bed do not exercise, study, or do other activities that stimulate the mind or body or emotions. Do not work too late at night. Avoid stimulants and spicy or stimulating food at night. Warm milk before bed can be relaxing, as can melatonin. You can also try chamomile tea, or tea with valerian in it. A warm, relaxing bath before bed is also a nice idea. People who get more sleep than they need will not fall asleep quickly at night. Avoid excess sleep or daytime naps.

Environment

Have a peaceful sleeping environment. A bit of fresh air in the room is nice if possible. Control the sound. Wear earplugs if you have to. Have clean, comfortable sheets. Use the right pillow for you. Make your sleeping space as conducive as possible to deep, healing sleep.

HYPNOTIC SUGGESTIONS

Verbal

I sleep deeply and soundly. I focus on my body when I go to sleep, noticing the feelings of heaviness and relaxation. My body is comfortable and heavy; my mind is quiet. I sleep deeply, feeling refreshed and relaxed when I awaken. I am going to awaken in the morning feeling great, I slept so deeply. I can see myself falling deeply asleep. My mind is quiet now. Nothing is important now. Peace is all that I feel. Everything in my life is going to work out perfectly. I trust in the perfection of life. I know that life is sometimes a mystery. I have no need to know all the answers to my questions now. I am at peace, knowing that everything that I need will come to me in time. I am at peace. I am falling into a deeply peaceful sleep.

Visual

See yourself being very heavy like a rock, sinking down into your bed. You are falling asleep, having a very hard time keeping your eyes open. Imagine that it is the next morning and the sun is coming in through the windows. You are waking up looking very, very happy and feeling refreshed, relaxed, and peaceful. You are smiling, stretching. You start to sing and laugh. You are happy to be alive. You are confident. You know that everything is going to be fine. You see yourself looking confident and more powerful than ever before. You look very happy and completely rested.

Metaphoric

Be a heavy rock sinking down in warm, soft sand. Be butter melting of top of hot oatmeal. Become the hibernating bear.

PERSONAL PLANS

_____

_____

_____

_____

_____

_____

_____

_____

Learning

ACTION LAYERS

Person

A relaxed mind-body state is more conducive to rapid learning than a tense one. Clear your mind of obstructive thoughts. Hold a positive attitude about learning, loving to learn new things. Allow yourself to be curious again. Throw away the fear of failure. Find what you love in the learning, and remember its place within your larger goals. Let learning be fun. A calm mind and body learn more. Try tai chi, yoga, or meditation.

Behavior

Have a time and place for study and practice, and focus on learning during that time. Discipline will pay off. Take time for relaxation and play too. Your mind will be clearer and your energy more focused if you have balance in your life. In Chinese medicine we recognize excess work as one of the causes of illness. There is nothing redeeming or altruistic about all work and no play; in ancient medicine that was considered unwise. It is your life, so have fun (but not too much) and do your work, as work gives meaning to life. Work hard, relax, and exercise—stay in balance. Be consistent in your studies. Long-term memory is best when you study and review regularly. Knowledge and skills build one step at a time. Do brief relaxation exercises right before you take exams. When you are in the exam room, do a one minute method body-mind relaxation. Review right before an exam as the content will be fresh in your memory.

Environment

Have a suitable learning environment. If the one you have is not suitable then find another one, get ear plugs, or do whatever else you need to do to make it work for you. You are unique, honor your unique needs. Associate with other focused, success-oriented individuals. Also, remember to eat healthy food. There are many brain foods on the market, like gingko biloba and gota kola. A vitamin supplement with B complex can also help with stress.

HYPNOTIC SUGGESTIONS

Verbal

I learn very, very quickly. The information flows into my mind and body and is absorbed completely. I easily recall and use this information when I need it. It is coming in perfectly. I am studying and practicing. I enjoy my study and practice time and look forward to it. I feel relaxed and clear minded when I learn. I am having fun. This is one of the best times of my life. It is my good fortune to have this chance to grow in knowledge, skills, and opportunity.

Visual

See yourself studying, very focused, looking serious, relaxed, and confident. See yourself taking the exam or doing the performance, and everything is smooth sailing. You look and feel great.

Metaphoric

Be a great library full of all of the information you need. Be a receptacle of knowledge and wisdom. Guardians move through the library keeping things in order, putting everything in the right place. They know exactly where to find what is needed whenever anyone asks for it. The guardians help you to find the things you need. They guide you in your search for skill and knowledge.

PERSONAL PLANS

_____

_____

_____

_____

_____

_____

_____

_____

_____

_____

_____

Pain

ACTION LAYERS

Person

Chronic physical pain can create emotional issues—anger, frustration, and depression. These will have to be addressed. Then of course there is the physical pain sensation. Hypnotic analgesia can help with this (see chapter 8). You will also want to work with relaxation. When the body has chronic pain, it can often create muscular tightening in the painful area in an effort to limit movement and discomfort. That tightening becomes a secondary source of pain, and it reduces flexibility causing other problems. Stay relaxed and upbeat as much as you can.

Behavior

Pain can produce secondary gain behaviors. This means that people's pain can be reinforcing because it gains the sufferer extra attention, access to drugs that can create dependence, and other dubious benefits. Secondary gains such as drugs and attention will reinforce the pain and make it harder to remove it. Any such secondary benefits will need to be examined and dealt with. Denial and false logic may present real challenges. The goal is to be as healthy and strong—physically, emotionally, and socially—as possible.

Environment

Use the resources in your environment that can help you, such as physical therapy, acupuncture and herbs, or massage. Be mindful when practitioners want you to get frequent X-rays, come back endlessly for treatment, or eagerly advise surgery or other expensive treatments. That often benefits them much more than it benefits you. Be a conscious consumer. Getting a second opinion in such cases can be very prudent. Seek reputable care. Become knowledgeable and more responsible for your own healing. Also, associate with positive, fun people.

HYPNOTIC SUGGESTIONS

Verbal

For pain: I am calm and relaxed. I feel the healing energy flowing through my body and through my pain. I love my body, and I work with it creatively and positively. My body feels great. My pain dissolves, and my body feels wonderful.

For secondary gains: I am free of artificial aids. I love myself and feel loved by the universe. I help myself. I take care of my needs, and I let others help me as needed. I am very independent and capable.

Visual

See yourself looking healthy, taking proactive steps to healing, being positive and strong. See yourself as happy and energetic.

Metaphoric

Become a tree. Trees are both strong and flexible. Work with metaphoric opposites. If the pain is cold, send it warm energy. If it is warm, send it cool energy. Ask your mind, "If the pain had a color, what color would it be?" Then ask your inner mind what the opposite, healing color would be. Send that healing color to the painful area over and over again. Speak to the pain and find out what it needs. When it answers through your inner mind, seek to give it the positive, healing things it needs.

Other Ideas

For specific pain, like headaches, menstrual cramps, or dental pain, relax and send cool or warm (depending on your need or preference) healing energy and a wonderful healing color to the area. Create hypnotic analgesia in your hand (so your hand becomes increasingly numb, chapter 8) and then place your hand on the area to transfer the analgesia to the pain directly. If you had dental work or some other type of surgery, you can suggest reduced swelling, rapid healing, healing energy flowing in the area, minimal pain, and good feelings. Pain can also be a signal of other things, such as more serious underlying issues or unresolved emotional concerns. If the pain persists see a medical professional to get an assessment. If the pain is a reflection of emotional issues, you may need to deal with the issue at the emotional (person) level for the problem to really heal. In that case, you may benefit from receiving professional counseling services.

PERSONAL PLANS

_____

_____

_____

_____

_____

_____

_____

_____

_____

_____

_____

_____

_____

Procrastination

ACTION LAYERS

Person

Fill your mind with enthusiasm for what you are doing. Talk yourself into an inspired state. Learn to relax, releasing any physical anxiety that may be obstructing you from taking action. Acknowledge any fear you have, and then do it, whatever it is. Practice being aware of when you are wasting time. Ask yourself why you are wasting time. If it is fear then move through it. Use self-hypnosis to regulate mental, emotional, or physical states that may be keeping you from doing your work. Banish negative, fearful thoughts. Bring in your courage, confidence, and power. Calm your emotions with breath. Quiet down your body. Whenever you find your wheels spinning, then just stop. Take a break. Do a quick refocusing session. If you still cannot work, then it is time to take a break. Enjoy it.

Behavior

Plan your day. Make a to-do list, prioritize it, check things off one at a time as you accomplish them. By planning every day, you give yourself focus and direction. Make a goal list for the week, month, and year, and check it as appropriate. Make sure your actions are in line with your long-term and short-term goals. Get excited about your life by embracing your goals and your dream. Make your activities part of your dream. Have fun.

Environment

Associate with positive, active, productive, successful people. Do not listen to the complainers. Run away from them as fast as you can. Go out and live your life now. Keep your to-do list easily accessible. Keep your environment organized. Place your things where they need to be for you to work effectively. Have your work-related resources available. Clear the surface of your work space. Remove clutter and other things that can distract you and waste your time. Keep your space simple and clean.

HYPNOTIC SUGGESTIONS

Verbal

I am proactive in my life. I go out and do what needs to be done. My goals are very important to me. I deserve to be happy. I take action because my actions are powerful, and they change the world in positive ways. No one else has my gifts but me. The world needs me to take action and make a difference. I love my life. I love this world. I take action now.

Visual

See yourself going for a full life and having fun. See yourself being passionate and intense, believing in your dream and doing it. If you currently have to do something that is not the ideal, then consider it a necessary stage you have to go through to get to your goal. Hold on to your dream. Imagine your dream as true.

Metaphoric

You are a steam engine going full speed ahead. Be an arrow heading straight for the bull's-eye or a powerful, charging animal. Be an immovable mountain, unshakeable, steadfast in your resolve.

PERSONAL PLANS

_____

_____

_____

_____

_____

_____

_____

_____

_____

_____

Relationships and Love

ACTION LAYERS

Person

Learn to relax. Remove negative, self-critical thoughts from your mind. Install positive attitudes about loving yourself and others. Strongly embrace the belief that you deserve to be loved and to be happy, and that you absolutely need to love yourself. Self-love is the beginning of strong, loving relationships. When we doubt our worthiness to be loved we collapse energetically. Believe that you are lovable. Bring in confidence and worthiness.

Behavior

Notice which behaviors attract people and which ones alienate people. Build the positive behaviors and reduce the negative ones. Mistakes and failures are inevitable, part of learning, part of being human. Keep at it. Love others and let them be who they are. People are doing the best they can at any moment given their resources and life experiences (and of course we can all do better). Let people be who they are, love them, and help them to be and do their best. Work on healing yourself. Communication is critically important. Communication is absolutely essential as a key to relationship happiness and success. The better you are at clearly stating your needs, asking for what you want, listening and seeking to understand others so their needs are met, the better your relationships will be. Giving and receiving are essential for any relationship. If you primarily give or receive, you are not in a balanced relationship. Learn how to give and receive real love.

Environment

Meeting: Go to places were you can meet people. Allow yourself time to be in those places; that is, do not go in the door then run away saying there is no one interesting inside. Join clubs or organizations where you can meet the kind of people you find interesting. Being alone, or being in places with the wrong type of people for you, will not lead to developing relationships.

Codependence: It takes two to tango. If you are being codependent so is the other person in your relationship. Both parties will need to work on the issue if any lasting change is going to occur. Observe healthy interpersonal relationships. Find an older, loving couple that is very successful in their relationship and see what they do. This can give you ideas about what effective loving relationships look like. If you find a genuinely loving couple, emulate them as much as is fitting for you. If you have a history of attracting destructive relationships, you may consider joining an appropriate 12-step group.

HYPNOTIC SUGGESTIONS
Verbal
I am a lovable and loving person. I attract other wonderful people into my life. I have good communication skills. I enjoy people. I am a lovable person just the way I am. People accept me for who I am, and I accept them. I love myself deeply. I attract whole, loving people into my life. I am a whole, loving person.

Visual
See yourself with friends or a loving partner. See the other person as someone you want in your life as a friend or partner—positive, encouraging, fun, successful. See yourself being happy whether you are with others or alone. Image yourself as encouraging others' growth, as feeling capable and independent, and as positively associating with good people.

Metaphoric
Like a magnet, become able to draw good things toward you. Be irresistible. Be strong and independent like a redwood tree, feeling that strength and flexibility. Imagine yourself being covered with a magical golden dust that makes you very attractive to other people. They sense your radiant, caring, positive energy. They want to come talk to you. You feel very confident when you put it on.

PERSONAL PLANS

_____

_____

_____

_____

_____

_____

_____

_____

_____

_____

Sales and Business

ACTION LAYERS

Person

Get inspired emotionally. Have a totally positive and persistent attitude. Know that you will succeed. Expect success. Be a winner in your mind. Know that you have the skills and qualities that it takes to succeed. Know that people believe in you. Banish negative thoughts. Banish fear. Build inner confidence. Deal with physical anxiety. Keep your emotions on an even keel. Take a steady course and keep moving higher. Know you are a winner. Stay highly motivated. Expect the best, recover quickly, do not let things keep you down. Keep rolling.

Behavior

Keep your energy up with a good diet and exercise. Look your best and emanate success. Send out a message of confidence and ability. Read motivational material. There are a lot of good books and courses on selling. The more you learn, the better. Keep refining your skills. Learn to really listen. Learn to pay attention. Chart your progess. Have a reward system. Do things that keep up your spirits and your motivation to succeed. Sing your success song every day.

Environment

Associate with positive and motivated individuals. Create an effective system for your work. Keep your work space and work materials organized. Have things where you need them to feel efficient. This will also help to build confidence. Streamline processes and work on improving everything that you do. Keep your goals foremost, goals for health, income, social, and family life. Work consistently on that dream.

HYPNOTIC SUGGESTIONS

Verbal

I love calling on clients. They are happy to speak with me, and we have a strong connection. They want to do business with me, and I want to support their success. I go the extra mile, and my clients want to work with me. I am extremely successful. My energy is very high, very strong. I take total responsibility for my outcomes, and I am a great success. I love my life.

Visual

See yourself making calls looking powerful, successful, and confident. See the other party being interested, smiling, asking questions, and signing contracts. See yourself closing sales and making deals. See the money growing in your bank account. See yourself carrying money into the bank in a wheelbarrow. You have growing resources to improve your life and the life of others.

Metaphoric

Be a bridge that spans the space between clients and the goods or services they need. The bridge is open, and the traffic will flow for years.

PERSONAL PLANS

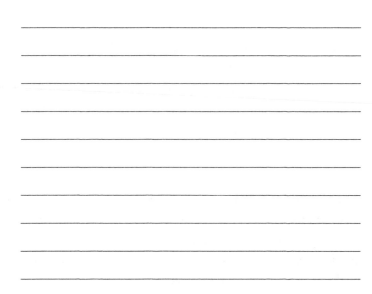

Self-Confidence, Shyness, and Self-Love

ACTION LAYERS

Person

Learn to relax deeply. Remove critical self-talk. Fill your mind with positive beliefs about yourself. You deserve to be happy. Remember that you are a learner, and you are learning new ways to be in the world. Shyness is very self-focused, self-protective. It is a fear of being hurt, a belief that we cannot be loved, that we are not good enough. Bringing in courage and confidence is very useful. Another strategy is to bring in awareness of others. Think about encouraging and loving them. This way of thinking automatically shifts attention away from self and can be very useful.

Behavior

Take good care of yourself. Treat yourself with respect. Praise yourself for having the courage to heal your past. Learn to forgive yourself and move on. Deal with denial and anger and hurt. Begin to focus on your gifts, your goals, and your dream. Take responsibility and action, and make your life wonderful. There is no one else in the world like you, no one. Learn to compliment others; building such generosity will make you more loved in the world, and that feedback will strengthen your courage to go forward. Learn to compliment yourself also. It is very important. World-class athletes do it all the time. Stretch yourself. Take some risks. Life is short. So what if someone says, "No thanks." Make it fun. It is not that big a deal. Let life be fun, more of a game.

Environment

Associate with people who respect you and who encourage your growth and self-love. If you are an introvert, do not expect to feel at home with a loud bunch of extroverts. They are not like you, so do not compare yourself to extroverts. Introverts will be less obvious at a party, but they will definitely be there, probably having a nice conversation with another introvert. Go find those people. You will recognize a commonality of energy. People are all different. Recognize and honor that. You do not have to be like anyone else but you.

HYPNOTIC SUGGESTIONS

Verbal

I love myself. I am a wonderful person. I am growing and learning every day. I learn new ways of being in the world. Life is great. Life is amazing. I feel totally confident, powerful, loved, and lovable. I want to share my gifts with the world. I love myself for who I am. I am having fun in my life. I feel more and more that life is an amazing adventure. I love playing with the possibilities, exploring life at every moment. Each day I wake up is another day to explore. I feel like I am on vacation, summer vacation. I can experience everything new. Life is great. People are great. I am having an amazing adventure.

Visual

See yourself as a confident, strong, and generous person. Imagine a guardian angel who comes and tells you the positive things you need to hear about yourself. You are generous, complimenting others in genuine ways. You are looking for ways to make others feel comfortable. You see other people are very relaxed and at ease with you, very interested in spending time with you.

Metaphoric

Be a precious child. Feel loved in the way very strong and kind parents would love and encourage their child. They want you to succeed. Be a warrior, strong and confident. Be an otter, having fun with life.

PERSONAL PLANS

_____

_____

_____

_____

_____

_____

_____

_____

_____

_____

_____

Sexual Health

ACTION LAYERS

Person

Relaxation is very helpful in improving sexual health. Your body has to learn to associate sexuality with pleasure, fun, and comfort. Relaxation is a good way to start. Banish negative thoughts about your body or your sexual ability. Just banish such useless garbage. Remove any comparisons with others; you are you. Patience and a noncritical attitude are essential. There is a good deal of confusion in our culture around sex because it has been made into such a commodity. Sex is really a simple thing. Let it be simple. Let it be pleasurable, fun, relaxing, and energizing. Let it be positive. It is about relationships with self, with other, and with spirit. Let it heal you.

Behavior

If your concern has more to do with sexual addictions then you should refer to the section on addictions. If you are troubled by some of your sexual behaviors or thoughts, it can be helpful to seek professional help. Our feelings and behaviors about sex are sometimes more common than we think, but they can still cause a lot of pain. There is no need for you to suffer. Regarding sexual performance, or function, trying to make things happen sexually is not the best strategy. Emphasize fun, not work. There is no need to hurry; why rush something pleasurable? Take your time. Make it enjoyable. Seek to make love, to generate more love. Ultimately that heals. Sexual healing is done through the mutual creation of love. Making love means to make love. Work with that concept. Explore it. This might include the need to improve relationships. Other things that greatly aid sexual healing are a high quality diet, supplements, tonic herbs, regular exercise, limited use of alcohol, and abstinence from cigarettes and marijuana.

Environment

It takes two to tango. Sexual issues can be the result of incompatibility, unresolved emotional issues, or a million other things. The cause needs to be examined. It can be beneficial to work with a therapist who deals with couples or sexual issues. Ultimately the goal is to create a sexual experience that is mutually fun and is an evolving loving experience. Get the information you need to help you understand your issue, such as books on sex therapy or tantra. There are lots of good resources out there. Tantric approaches allow you to work with sexuality on an energetic level that can be very helpful.

HYPNOTIC SUGGESTIONS

Verbal

I enjoy making love. Sexual energy is healing my body and spirit. It is wonderful to connect with another human heart in a deeply loving way. I love my body. I love who I am. My sexual energy flows easily. The energy heals me and the one I love. I love making love. I am having fun. I can feel my energy in every part of my body. Vitality is filling every part of my body. I feel incredible. It is so great to be alive. I love people. My heart is healing, and I can feel love more and more. I want my love to heal others. I want love to heal me. I feel more and more at peace. I know that healing is happening now.

Visual

See yourself being sexual in a healthy, fun, loving way. See yourself and your partner having fun. See your body looking fit, energetic, vital. See yourself as playful and healthy, turned on, happy to be alive. Imagine that you are a body of pure energy. Feel the energy coursing through you. Feel the energy building and flowing. Recognize the vast power of life flowing through you.

Metaphoric

For functional issues, be a drawbridge going up or a garden gate opening. For sexual play, be an animal. Otters have fun, lions are sexually intense. Be a volcano or an ocean wave.

Other Ideas

Although it is not common knowledge in our culture, there is an ancient art of lovemaking called tantra. In the East this body of knowledge has been used for centuries. Although the bulk of tantric work in the East is more typically energy work of a nonsexual nature, there is a sexual branch to the practice. Tantric sex work is gaining popularity in the West. You can find many good books on the subject written by Westerners. These books contain helpful ideas regarding working with sexual energy. It is a very powerful energy, which can be used for high spiritual purposes.

PERSONAL PLANS

_____

_____

_____

_____

_____

_____

_____

_____

_____

_____

_____

Skin Conditions

ACTION LAYERS

Person

Relaxation is very helpful in aiding skin conditions. Releasing anger and other negative emotions may also prove helpful in some cases. In Chinese medicine we often associate skin conditions with internal heat. Strong emotion can stagnate energy and generate such internal heat. Keep your emotions in balance, let go of your anger, and increase your gratitude. If physical anxiety or negative emotions cause you to eat poorly, then it is important to work on addressing those levels of the issue. Keep your body, mind, and spirit harmonious, positive, and happy.

Behavior

Determine whether any particular behaviors are related to your condition—such as inappropriate diet, stress, or not bathing every day—and work on that pattern. Try to pay attention to behavioral patterns that appear to be related to skin changes. Play with these patterns. Diet is very important. Watch what you eat. Oily foods, spicy foods, colas, and chocolate will often create acne and make other skin conditions worse. Try to eat greens and more vegetables; see what happens. Eat healthy, fresh foods. Avoid junk food. You deserve good things. Also, clip the stressors in your life. Relax more.

Environment

Determine what environmental factors may be stimulating or increasing your reaction. Many substances in the environment can be highly irritating and allergenic. This can include makeup, chemicals in body products, ingredients in foods, or materials in the workplace. Reduce your contact with these agents if you begin to recognize reactivity. See if it improves with reduced contact. Also, toxic social environments can stress the body-mind. See if you can mitigate their influence. Let the world work for you, not against you.

HYPNOTIC SUGGESTIONS

Verbal

I am very happy and take responsibility for my attitudes. They are very positive. My skin is smooth and soft. It is becoming healthier and healthier. My skin looks and feels very healthy. I feel great. I love how I look. I eat the right foods that balance my body chemistry and my skin. I take care of my health, and my energy is strong. My mind is calm, and my body is clean. I feel great.

Visual

See your skin becoming more and more balanced and nonreactive. Your skin appears smooth, your eyes are clear and bright, other signs of balance are evident. See yourself looking happy and healthy. Use counter imagery: if the condition is hot and dry then imagine cool, softening energy flowing through the specific affected area. If a skin patch is red, hot, and itchy then select an ideal antidote temperature, color, and feeling, and visualize that energy in the problem location. It can be a very simple and helpful strategy.

Metaphoric

Be the smooth surface of still, cool water. Be the water. Become the clear blue sky. Become a cooling, cleansing summer rain. Be smooth like satin. Be a baby again, with baby soft skin.

PERSONAL PLANS

Sports and Performance

ACTION LAYERS

Person

Use a lot of positive self-talk and positive visual imagery. Bring in powerful positive attitudes and beliefs for your success. Develop strong, positive expectations about your performance. Learn how to relax deeply and quickly, and bring that relaxation into your performance to increase your sense of flow. Keep your body calm, your mind focused and still, and your emotions positive. Make your inner system work for you, support you. Be confident, believing in yourself. Have a strong positive expectation. You will succeed.

Behavior

Practice consciously with the intention of noticing your patterns and removing what is inefficient or ineffective and increasing what works best. Eat well, get rest, and take care of your body to avoid injuries and to be able to perform your best. Eat for energy. Eat for nutrients. If you eat for nutrients, your diet will be clean and empowering. Eat to feel power. Avoid pesticides and food additives. Get fresh air, and drink clean water. Stay organized and manage your time well so that can reduce stress from excess demands on your time. Use your time well. Be efficient and productive. Make it all count.

Environment

Associate with people who are as good as or better than you at your sport or performance area. Learn from them. Find someone who is the best at what you want to do. Watch videos of them, follow their game, become them, emulate their swing, serve, steps. Try to find out how they train, what they eat, how they practice, what their mental game is like. Become that person, and then integrate the essence of what makes them effective and toss out the idiosyncratic elements of their style. Feel what they feel, see what they see, think what they think. Once it is in you, it is yours. Then you can integrate and incorporate their lessons into your unique style.

HYPNOTIC SUGGESTIONS

Verbal

I am excellent at _____. My mind and body are totally focused when I do _____. Every ounce of my energy is channeled into an excellent performance. I love doing _____. I am a powerful athlete/performer. I love what I do. It gives me such a sense of joy. I seek to be the best I can be in this area. I am developing my body, mind, and spirit. I am totally confident when I perform. I feel solid, absolutely solid. I know I will succeed. The audience is so supportive. I feel their support and that energy helps me to fly. I feel incredible. My body is strong. My mind is clear. My heart is happy and powerful. I know I will succeed. I feel great.

Visual

Always rehearse in your mind. Practice doing pieces of the action perfectly in your mind and get ideas about how to be even better. Always see the peak sports performance in your visual imagery. See yourself doing an element of the game/match/performance excellently. Break it down into components when necessary; perfect weaker areas. Practice the whole process as well, if applicable. At times, include the appropriate audience as part of your mental rehearsal. See the crowd going wild in support of your performance. Feel the energy flowing through your body. You are intense and powerful.

Metaphoric

Be a laser of focused power, a powerful animal, an incredibly finely tuned machine, a radiant being moved by a divine force.

PERSONAL PLANS

_____

_____

_____

_____

_____

_____

_____

_____

_____

_____

Weight Management

ACTION LAYERS

Person

Have a positive attitude about your body and your ability to manage your weight. Know you will succeed in your goals. Give up on becoming some perfect weight. Get in shape and your natural ideal will become apparent. Love yourself. Have an upbeat outlook. Deal with depression, anger, and other burdensome emotions. Keep your emotions calm and steady. Stay positive as much as possible. Become a problem solver. Know that you have a great power within yourself to succeed. Allow yourself to be a success. Weight is often not the only issue, self-love is often a problem too. Work on both, and you will be exponentially healthy. Believe in yourself, love yourself, be yourself.

Behavior

Eat healthy—lower in fat, higher in protein and complex carbohydrates. Avoid fad diets. Exercise is also a key ingredient to successful weight management. Make exercise something fun, part of an enjoyable way to be healthy. Think of your health, with weight management being just one part of a bigger picture. Make the process pleasurable. Eat for nutrients, not for caloric content. Eat green, natural, and organic. Avoid pesticides, genetically altered foods, additives, sweeteners, artificial substances, and processed foods. Learn how to cook. Make that a fun thing. Make that a positive social experience.

Environment

Avoid eating at places that serve unhealthy foods. Keep your house free of inappropriate foods. Join a club or find other fun places to exercise.

Find a place to exercise. Find an exercise partner. Make a plan and implement it. If it is helpful, join a group that assists people with eating and weight management. Get the books that you need or other resources. Take positive action. Associate with positive, affirming people.

HYPNOTIC SUGGESTIONS

Verbal

I love my body. I am healthy, energetic, and happy. I am at the ideal weight for my body. I feel great. I am so happy to be alive. I take such good care of myself. I eat right, exercise, drink fresh water, associate with loving people, read inspirational materials. I love my life. I have a strong desire to only eat healthy foods, to eat moderately, and to move my body. I have a tremendous capacity to accomplish my goals. I am excited about life. I look forward to getting up every morning and starting my day. My life is incredible. I feel great. My body is strong, flexible, vital, and alive. I love my body. I love myself. I love this life.

Visual

See yourself as fit, healthy, and energetic. You are doing active exercise and having fun. You are eating healthy food and loving the energy it gives you. See a radiant body of energy. You are like the sun. Warm, radiant light is coming from you. You feel that energy. It fills you with joy and peace. It is melting away sluggish, sticky energy. See yourself running with the wind. You are light and free. You feel fresh air on your face. The fragrance is uplifting. You have angel wings, and you are being carried up by the warm drafts of a summer breeze. You are light, soaring. You can see beautiful hills below. You fly to a special garden. There you are met by great healers. You sit in the garden with them. You feel their healing energy flowing into you. You are strong, peaceful, healthy; you feel wonderful, and you look great.

Metaphoric

Be powerful and physical, toned like a jaguar. You are a hillside covered with snow. The warm spring sun is melting away the layers of snow. Vital new life is rising up. The winter has ended. Spring is here.

PERSONAL PLANS

_____

_____

_____

_____

_____

_____

_____

_____

_____

_____

_____

_____

_____

final thoughts

This book is designed to be a useful resource in developing a personal self-hypnosis practice. Healing, self-improvement, learning a new skill, and increasing personal performance are not occasional events. They all require diligent practice and persistence. The more vigilant you are with them, the faster your personal progress will be. It is my hope that you will actively employ the methods outlined in this book to make your life more and more incredible. As these hypnotic tools become more internalized, you will be able to access your inherent capacity for unlimited change and growth.

It is time to say farewell for now. When letting go of a hand or sharing a final word, there arrives a moment of wonder. In that deep space, in that essential stillness, if we look between the lines of time and place, we can see without hesitation the vast field of hypnotic dreams where all meetings are eternally possible. I hope your life affords you the chance to work with these new transformational skills and to develop confidence with them. Hypnosis is a special gift. It is a key that opens up a secret world. It allows us to enter that deep space within our beings where we can explore the vast potentials of this experience called life. For those who find that key, the adventures are great. So the best of luck to you on your journeys. Remember to keep the light on in your heart; it will help you to find your way home. And wherever you go, may your learnings bring the greatest peace and happiness to you and to our planet. Until next time.

index

ideomotor behavior, 77
inducing hypnosis with, 57
posthypnotic suggestion, 77, 88-89, 100
proprioceptive distortion, 77-78
time distortion, 71, 78
Hypnotic state
benefits of, 25-26
depth of, 32-33
indications of, 58
inducing, 53-54
sleep versus, 66
Hypnotic suggestions. *See also* Verbal suggestions; Visual suggestions
affirmations versus, 83-84
direct suggestion, 57, 66
effortfulness of, 82-83
metaphoric, 95-96, 97, 110
samples of, 96-97
transforming beliefs and, 37, 81-82

I

Ideomotor behavior, 77
Imagery. *See* Visual imagery
Incompetence, 10
Induction methods. *See also* Focusing
attention fixation, 56
direct suggestion, 57, 66
fused eyelids, 60, 71-72, 75, 104, 108
heavy hand, 61
hypnotic phenomena for, 57
inner focus, 54-55
look up, hold, drop down, 59
magnetic hands, 57, 60-61, 77
mental imagery and absorption, 56
overview, 36-37, 53-54
repetitive stimuli, 55
Inertia, 11-12
Infants, 3-4
Inner focus induction, 54-55
Inner peace, 59
Inner wisdom, 34
Insomnia, 65, 136-138. *See also* Sleep
Introverts versus extroverts, 149
Intuition, 19, 25

L

Lasers, 41
Learning. *See also* Mind-body learning
clarifying goals and, 21
dreamlike states and, 25
effortless, 82
feedback for, 41
focusing attention and, 22
hypnosis session for, 138-140

relearning beliefs, 16-17
theta brain waves during, 23-24
vicarious, 25-26
Left brain, 18, 19, 22, 24-25
Letting go, 59
Light sphere, 70
Limiting beliefs
awareness of, 7-9
conscious mind and, 83
cultural beliefs as, 7-8
family beliefs as, 8
inertia and, 11-12
maintaining, 9-12, 23
problem with, 5-6
as self-fulfilling, 12-13
self-identity and, 3-4
self-protective nature of, 16
thoughts and, 23, 94
transforming or removing, 13
Location for hypnosis sessions, 35-36
Logic, 8-9, 18
Look up, hold, drop down induction, 59
Love, 145-147. *See also* Self-love

M

Magnetic hands, 57, 60-61, 77
Mandala, 56
Meditation, 23, 24, 26, 54
Memories, 73
Menstrual cramps, 142
Mental imagery induction, 56
Metaphoric suggestions, 95-96, 97, 110
Metronome, 67
Mind-body energy field, 82
Mind-body learning. *See also* Learning
approaches to, 15-16
Eastern perspective, 19
hypnosis and, 20
left and right brain and, 18-19
relearning beliefs, 16-17
Money, 33-34, 87. *See also* Prosperity
Music, 55
Mythology, 95

N

Nail biting, 27. *See also* Habit control
Negative beliefs, 2, 5-6. *See also* Limiting
beliefs
Negative thoughts, 34, 94
New ideas, 25

O

Ocean of bliss, 70
One minute method, 28-29, 50